ONE STOP DOC
Cardiovascular System

One Stop Doc

Titles in the series include:

Cell and Molecular Biology – Desikan Rangarajan and David Shaw
Editorial Advisor – Barbara Moreland

Gastrointestinal System – Miruna Canagaratnam
Editorial Advisor – Richard Naftalin

Nervous System – Elliott Smock
Editorial Advisor – Clive Coen

Coming soon...

Respiratory System – Jo Dartnell and Michelle Ramsay
Editorial Advisor – John Rees

Musculoskeletal System – Bassel Zebian and Wayne Lam
Editorial Advisor – Alistair Hunter

Renal System and Electrolyte Balance – Panos Stamoulos and Spyros Bakalis
Editorial Advisors – Richard Naftalin and Alistair Hunter

Endocrine and Reproductive Systems – Caroline Jewel and Alexandra Tillett
Editorial Advisor – Stuart Milligan

Nutrition and Metabolism – Miruna Canagaratnam and David Shaw
Editorial Advisors – Barbara Moreland and Richard Naftalin

ONE STOP DOC

Cardiovascular System

Jonathan Aron BSc(Hons)
Fourth year medical student, Guy's, King's and
St Thomas' Medical School, London, UK

Editorial Advisor: Jeremy PT Ward PhD
Professor of Respiratory Cell Physiology, Department of Asthma
Allergies and Respiratory Medicine, Kings College, London, UK

Series Editor: Elliott Smock BSc(Hons)
Fifth year medical student, Guy's, King's and
St Thomas' Medical School, London, UK

ARNOLD

A member of the Hodder Headline Group
LONDON

First published in Great Britain in 2004 by
Arnold, a member of the Hodder Headline Group,
338 Euston Road, London NW1 3BH

http://www.arnoldpublishers.com

Distributed in the United States of America by
Oxford University Press Inc.,
198 Madison Avenue, New York, NY10016
Oxford is a registered trademark of Oxford University Press

British Library Cataloguing in Publication Data
A catalogue record for this book is available from the British Library

Library of Congress Cataloging-in-Publication Data
A catalog record for this book is available from the Library of Congress

ISBN 0 340 812508

1 2 3 4 5 6 7 8 9 10

Commissioning Editor: Georgina Bentliff
Project Editor: Heather Smith
Production Controller: Lindsay Smith
Cover Design: Amina Dudhia

Typeset in 10/12pt Adobe Garamond/Akzidenz GroteskBE by Servis Filmsetting Ltd, Manchester
Printed and bound in Spain

Hodder Headline's policy is to use papers that are natural, renewable and recyclable products
and made from wood grown in sustainable forests. The logging and manufacturing processes
are expected to conform to the environmental regulations of the country of origin.

What do you think about this book? Or any other Arnold title?
Please send your comments to **feedback.arnold@hodder.co.uk**

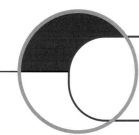

CONTENTS

PREFACE

From the Series Editor, Elliott Smock

Are you ready to face your looming exams? If you have done loads of work, then congratulations; we hope this opportunity to practice SAQs, EMQs, MCQs and Problem-based Questions on every part of the core curriculum will help you consolidate what you've learnt and improve your exam technique. If you don't feel ready, don't panic – the One Stop Doc series has all the answers you need to catch up and pass.

There are only a limited number of questions an examiner can throw at a beleaguered student and this text can turn that to your advantage. By getting straight into the heart of the core questions that come up year after year and by giving you the model answers you need, this book will arm you with the knowledge to succeed in your exams. Broken down into logical sections, you can learn all the important facts you need to pass without having to wade through tons of different textbooks when you simply don't have the time. All questions presented here are 'core'; those of the highest importance have been highlighted to allow even sharper focus if time for revision is running out. In addition, to allow you to organize your revision efficiently, questions have been grouped by topic, with answers supported by detailed integrated explanations.

On behalf of all the One Stop Doc authors I wish you the very best of luck in your exams and hope these books serve you well!

From the Author, Jonathan Aron

This book will make you experts in cardiovascular physiology. Probably. If not then at least it will prepare you for an exam on the subject. The book takes you on a quick tour of all of the important topics you'll find in the exam, and gives you exam experience. In addition, it is a textbook containing vital information needed for understanding a topic and key facts that you will be expected to know.

Cardiovascular physiology, in particular, is based on an understanding of key principles and once these have been learnt, any questions on the topic will be a doddle. The cardiovascular system comprises the heart and the vasculature. The heart has its own blood supply and has an electrical system to make sure it works properly. Thus this book is split into the following chapters: Vasculature, Blood supply to the heart, Heart, and Conduction of the heart. Logical, I hope you agree. The diagrams are all easily reproducible but still representative of the underlying complex scientific principles, so they can be scribbled down during an exam to help you visualise a problem. The book also includes some case studies so that the physiology and pharmacology you are learning has some relevance to your future clinical studies, and doesn't seem like a complete waste of time. And they are quite interesting . . .

I hope you'll find this book helpful. You may even develop an interest in the subject (or at the very least, a mild tolerance). Enjoy.

The whole lengthy process of writing and illustrating this book has been supervised by a cleverer man than myself, Professor Jeremy Ward, so many thanks to him are in order. He has supervised every stage, gone over every question and questioned every diagram until he was happy, so many thanks to him for all his help and patience over the last two years. Also thank you to Elliott who got me involved in this project. My parents (and brother) would kill me if I didn't include them here. And thanks to Chris and Wayne for offering criticism (not necessarily positive or relevant).

ABBREVIATIONS

ACE	angiotensin-converting enzyme
ACh	acetylcholine
ADH	antidiuretic hormone
ADP	adenosine diphosphate
AF	atrial fibrillation
AngI	angiotensin I
AngII	angiotensin II
ASD	atrial septal defect
ATP	adenosine triphosphate
AV node	atrioventricular node
AV	aortic valve
BP	blood pressure
cAMP	cyclic adenosine monophosphate
CK	creatine kinase
CO	cardiac output
COPD	chronic obstructive pulmonary disease
CT	computed tomography
CVP	central venous pressure
DAD	delayed after depolarization
DVT	deep vein thrombosis
EAD	early after depolarization
ECG	electrocardiogram
EDP	end diastolic pressure
EDV	end diastolic volume
EEL	external elastic lamina
ESV	end systolic volume
HDL	high density lipoprotein
HR	heart rate
IEL	internal elastic lamina
IP3	inositol-(1,4,5)-trisphosphate
IVC	inferior vena cava
JVP	jugular venous pressure
LCC	left common carotid
LDH	lactate dehydrogenase
LDL	low density lipoprotein
LHF	left heart failure
LSA	left subclavian artery
LV	left ventricle
Mj	macrophage
MI	myocardial infarction
MV	mitral valve
NO	nitric oxide
PE	pulmonary embolism
PGH_2	prostaglandin H_2
PGI_2	prostacyclin
PKA	protein kinase A
PKG	protein kinase G
PLD	phospholipase D
RA	right atrium
RBC	red blood cell
RCC	right common carotid
RSA	right subclavian artery
RV	right ventricle
SA node	sinoatrial node
SR	sarcoplasmic reticulum
SV	stroke volume
SVC	superior vena cava
SVT	supraventricular tachycardia
TA	tunica adventitia
TI	tunica intima
TM	tunica media
tPA	tissue plasminogen activators
Trop T	troponin T
TXA_2	thromboxane A_2
VF	ventricular fibrillation
VOCC	voltage-operated Ca^{2+} channel
VSD	ventricular septal defect
WPW	Wolff–Parkinson–White

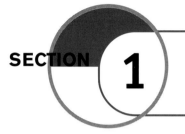

THE VASCULAR SYSTEM

1 ✓ THE VASCULAR SYSTEM

1. Consider the common blood vessels in the body. Put the following in order, starting with the vessel lumen of largest diameter and ending with the smallest

    A. Muscular artery
    B. Arteriole
    C. Vena cava
    D. Venule
    E. Ascending aorta
    F. Capillary
    G. Vein

2. Regarding blood vessels

FALSE   **a.** The wall thickness of the vena cava is greater than the aorta
TRUE   **b.** The capillary wall is 1 μm thick
FALSE   **c.** Arterial and venous anastomoses are widespread throughout the circulation
FALSE   **d.** Veins of the upper limbs contain semilunar valves
TRUE   **e.** Veins and arteries typically run together to conserve heat and aid venous return

3. True or false?

F **a.** The pulmonary circulation is driven by the left side of the heart
T **b.** The pulmonary trunk splits into the right and left pulmonary arteries
F **c.** The blood supply to the lungs is derived from intercostal arteries from the aorta
T **d.** The aorta terminates by splitting into the right and left common iliacs
F **e.** The abdominal aorta gives rise to the femoral artery

4. Which of the following is the false statement?

    a. Arterial anastomoses provide collateral circulation which is a means of alternative blood supply in times of ischaemia
  ✳**b.** The liver's main blood supply is derived from the hepatic artery
    c. The aortic arch gives rise to vessels supplying the head and arms
    d. The inferior vena cava drains blood returning from the abdomen and lower limbs into the right heart

---

*MI, myocardial infarction

EXPLANATION: ANATOMY OF THE VASCULAR SYSTEM

The gross anatomy of the vascular system is detailed below. The venous vessels tend to have larger lumens than their related arteries (i.e. vena cava > aorta and venules > arterioles). Arterial wall thickness, however, is greater.

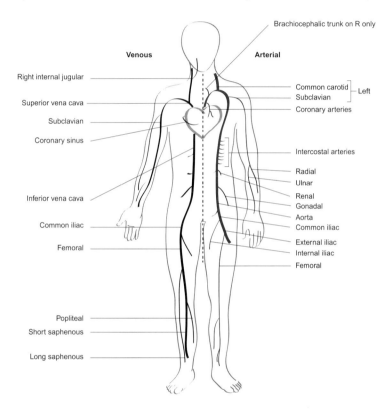

The right heart pumps blood through the pulmonary circulation, back into the left heart whose job it is to supply oxygenated blood to the rest of the body. This is done via the aorta, which supplies the myocardium (via the **coronary circulation**), the head and neck (via the **carotids** and **subclavian arteries**), the chest wall (via the **intercostal arteries**), and abdominal viscera. The exception to the rule is the liver, which receives 70 per cent of its blood supply from the portal vein and only 30 per cent from the hepatic artery. ✳

Other important facts to know are that veins in the lower limbs contain **semilunar valves** to prevent back flow and pooling of blood due to gravity. Arterial anastomoses such as in the heart may provide an alternative supply of blood if the usual supply is cut off (e.g. MI).

Answers

1. 1 – C, 2 – E, 3 – G, 4 – A, 5 – D, 6 – B, 7 – F
2. F T F F T
3. F T F T F
4. b

5. **Use the options below to label the diagram of a muscular artery**

Options

A. Vasa vajorum   B. Nerve bundle
C. Tunica adventitia   D. Tunica intima
E. Tunica media   F. Internal elastic lamina
G. External elastic lamina   H. Endothelial cells

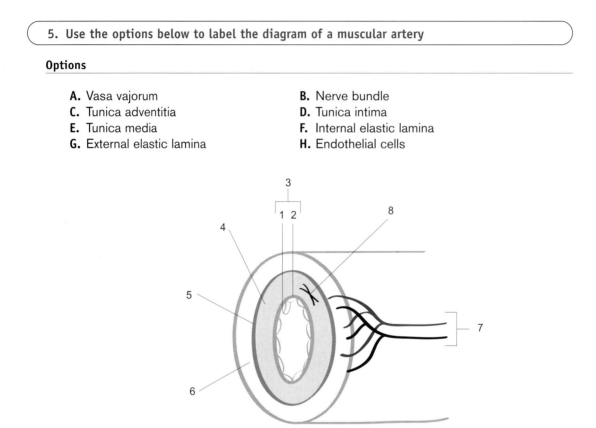

6. **Answer true or false regarding the endothelial layer**

F **a.** It is structurally similar to squamous epithelium
T **b.** The endothelium completely lines the insides of all blood vessels and lymphatics
T **c.** The blood–brain barrier contains continuous endothelium, which is impermeable to large molecules
F **d.** The kidneys and the liver circulation contain discontinuous endothelium
T **e.** The endothelium has an anticlotting effect

---

*TA, tunica adventitia; TM, tunica media; TI, tunica intima; IEL, internal elastic lamina; EEL, external elastic lamina; RBC, red blood cell

EXPLANATION: VASCULAR MICROSTRUCTURE

The figure below shows the microstructure of three different large vessels. Veins have the same three basic layers as arteries but they are less well-demarcated and the tunica media (TM) is thinner, with fewer smooth muscle cells. Smooth muscle is discussed on page 59.

From the innermost layer, outwards:

- **Endothelium** is a one-cell-thick layer. The cells are sealed to each other by tight junctions (unlike squamous epithelium), which modify vascular permeability, cell migration into the periphery and vasoconstriction
- **Tunica intima** (TI) consists of endothelium + connective tissue layer (the internal elastic lamina)
- **Internal elastic lamina** (IEL) consists of a dense elastic matrix
- **Tunica media** (TM) is the main part of the wall. In muscular arteries it contains elastin and circulatory smooth muscle so when the muscle contracts the lumen is narrowed. Veins contain more elastin and less smooth muscle. This is attached to the **external elastic lamina** (EEL)
- **Tunica adventitia** (TA) is the external 'coat' composed of connective tissue. It contains elastin and collagen
- **Blood supply** (vasa vajorum) and the **nerve bundle** infiltrates the tunica media.

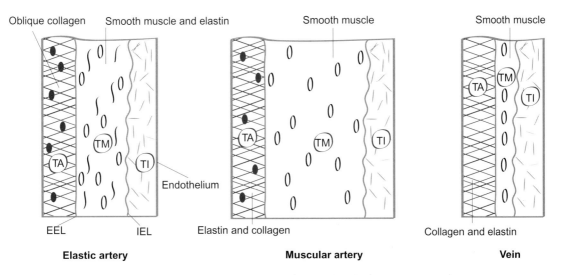

| **Elastic artery** | **Muscular artery** | **Vein** |

The endothelium has a number of important functions. It completely lines the inside of the vascular system (and lymphatics) and regulates permeability, clotting and immune function. There are three types: **continuous** (found in the blood–brain barrier and impermeable to large molecules), **fenestrated** (found in the liver, endocrine glands and kidneys and with numerous holes to allow molecules to cross) and **discontinuous** (found in the spleen, allowing RBCs to pass out of the circulation).

Answers
5. 1 – H, 2 – F, 3 – D, 4 – E, 5 – G, 6 – C, 7 – A, 8 – B
6. F T T F T

7. True or false? Nitric oxide

T **a.** Is manufactured and released by endothelial cells
T **b.** Is synthesized via the L-arginine nitric oxide synthase pathway
T **c.** Requires Ca^{2+} in its synthesis
f **d.** Causes smooth muscle contraction
f **e.** Has its action potentiated by superoxide anion

8. Which of the following act on the endothelium indirectly to cause smooth muscle contraction?

f **a.** Bradykinin
T **b.** Angiotensin II
T **c.** Thrombin
f **d.** Acetylcholine
f **e.** Adenosine diphosphate

9. Which of the following substances manufactured by the endothelial cell cause relaxation?

T **a.** Nitric oxide
f **b.** Superoxide anion
f **c.** Endothelin
T **d.** Prostacyclin
f **e.** Thromboxane A_2

10. Which of the following can be caused by endothelial dysfunction?

T **a.** Atheromatous plaque formation
T **b.** Thrombosis formation
T **c.** Hypertension
f **d.** Vascular shock
T **e.** Pre-eclampsia

---

*MI, myocardial infarction; NO, nitric oxide; TXA_2, thromboxane A_2; PGH_2, prostaglandin H_2; ACh, acetylcholine; AngII, angiotensin II; ADP, adenosine diphosphate; PGI_2, prostacyclin; PKG, protein kinase G; PKA, protein kinase A; ATP, adenosine triphosphate; cAMP, cyclic adenosine monophosphate

EXPLANATION: THE ENDOTHELIUM

The endothelium is responsible for maintaining **vascular tone**, providing **selective permeability**, regulating **inflammatory responses**, maintaining **thrombo-resistance** and guiding **vascular growth**. Diabetes mellitus causes endothelial damage as a result of abnormally high glucose levels in the bloodstream. This leads to hypertension, increased risk of arteriosclerosis and associated complications (coronary artery disease, blindness, etc.) and increased risk of MI due to abnormal clotting. Hypertension also contributes to endothelial dysfunction. (Which comes first? Chicken and egg dilemma.)

Vascular tone is maintained by **sympathetic**, **parasympathetic** and **humoral** control. In addition, metabolites alter tone (e.g. increase in CO_2 causes vasodilatation). The endothelium regulates hormonal control. Relaxing and contracting factors produced by the endothelium act on adjacent smooth muscle. PGH_2 causes vasoconstriction, as does TXA_2 and endothelin-1. Relaxing factors are PGI_2 and NO. Superoxide anion destroys NO, thus decreasing relaxation (= contraction). Bradykinin, ACh, adrenaline, prostaglandins and ADP in the blood cause release of relaxing factors, whereas AngII, thrombin, serotonin and noradrenaline cause release of contracting factors.

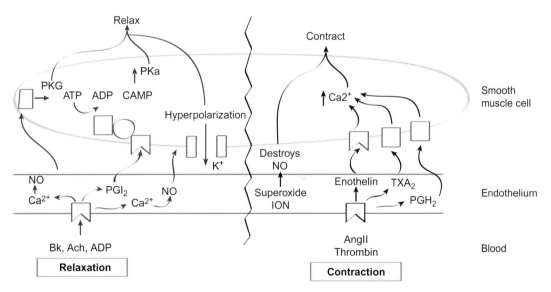

From Aaronson, Pl., Ward, J., Wiener, C.M., *The Cardiovascular System at a Glance*, 2nd edn, 2003. Redrawn with kind permission of Blackwell Science Ltd.

Answers
7. T T T F F
8. F T T F F
9. T F F T F
10. T T T F T

11. True or false? Baroreceptors

T **a.** Are found in the arch of the aorta and the carotid sinus
F **b.** Are innervated via sympathetic nerves
T **c.** Increase their output during systole
F **d.** Play an important role in long-term blood pressure regulation
T **e.** Modify vascular tone and heart rate when stimulated

12. True or false?

T **a.** Chemoreceptors are found in the periphery
T **b.** Chemoreceptors modulate the vasomotor centre of the brain
T **c.** Chemoreceptors are stimulated by an increase in CO_2 and H^+
F **d.** Central chemoreceptors respond to a decrease in O_2
T **e.** The vasomotor centre affects blood pressure by modifying sympathetic and parasympathetic outputs

13. Below is a flow diagram representing BP control by the kidney. Fill in the missing boxes with the options provided

Options

A. Angiotensin II
B. Vasoconstriction
C. Renal salt and water retention
D. Renin
E. Angiotensin-converting enzyme (ACE)
F. Aldosterone
G. Increased blood pressure
H. Decreased blood pressure

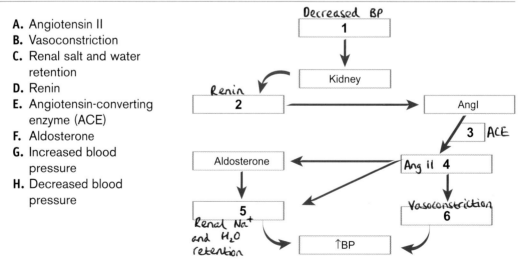

*BP, blood pressure; HR, heart rate; AngI, angiotensin I

EXPLANATION: CONTROL OF BLOOD PRESSURE

Short-term BP is monitored and controlled by **baroreceptors** found in the **arch of the aorta** and **carotid sinus**. These measure stretch of the arterial wall. If the wall starts to stretch because of increased pressure in the artery, vagal afferent impulses increase in frequency and vascular tone is reduced by decreasing sympathetic stimulation and increasing vagal (parasympathetic) stimulation, thus causing vasodilatation and drop in BP. HR is also modified: increased by increasing sympathetic drive and decreasing vagal drive or decreased by increasing vagal drive. Baroreceptors are useless at long-term BP control because they reset to whatever pressure they are exposed to for 1–2 days.

Central chemoreceptors respond to an increase in blood CO_2 (which dissociates to H^+). **Peripheral chemoreceptors** in addition respond to low levels of blood O_2.

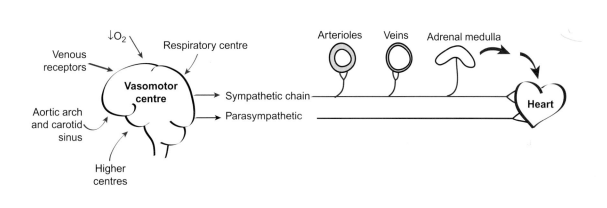

The single most important organ involved in long-term BP control is the **kidney**. BP in the renal artery regulates renin release, which activates the **renin-angiotensin-aldosterone** pathway. This is shown opposite. Atrial natriuretic peptide is released from the atria of the heart in response to atrial stretch (secondary to increased blood volume) and also acts on the kidney to increase water excretion.

Answers
11. T F T F T
12. T T T F T
13. 1 – H, 2 – D, 3 – E, 4 – A, 5 – C, 6 – B

14. Considering exercise

    a. A healthy person undertakes moderate exercise. Name three adaptive mechanisms the body employs to meet the increased energy requirements

    b. Name four methods of flow control in the capillary network

    c. During exercise, in which part of the body would you expect to find increased blood flow and where would you expect decreased blood flow?

    d. In which part of the vascular system does the greatest pressure drop occur?
    arterioles

15. Upon exercise, which of the three scenarios below is most likely to occur in:

Options

    A. A healthy individual? **3**
    B. A person in heart failure? **2**
    C. An elderly individual? **1**

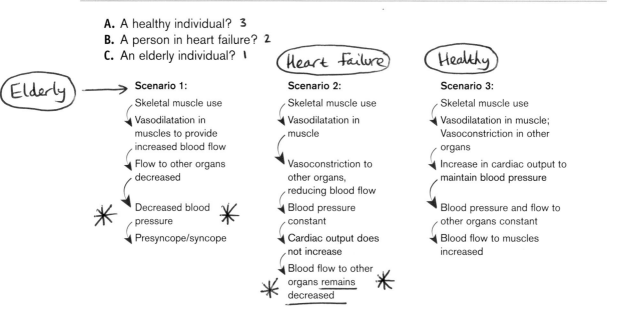

(Elderly) ──→ **Scenario 1:** *(Heart Failure)* **Scenario 2:** *(Healthy)* **Scenario 3:**

Scenario 1:	Scenario 2:	Scenario 3:
Skeletal muscle use	Skeletal muscle use	Skeletal muscle use
Vasodilatation in muscles to provide increased blood flow	Vasodilatation in muscle	Vasodilatation in muscle; Vasoconstriction in other organs
Flow to other organs decreased	Vasoconstriction to other organs, reducing blood flow	Increase in cardiac output to maintain blood pressure
Decreased blood pressure	Blood pressure constant	Blood pressure and flow to other organs constant
Presyncope/syncope	Cardiac output does not increase	Blood flow to muscles increased
	Blood flow to other organs remains decreased	

    D. What symptom is likely to be experienced by a person in heart failure?
    Shortness of breath

---

*CO, cardiac output; BP, blood pressure; HR, heart rate; SV, stroke volume

$$CO = HR \times SV$$

EXPLANATION: THE EFFECTS OF EXERCISE ON THE CIRCULATION

First, it is important to remember that the cardiovascular system is closed with a single pump driving the whole thing. Therefore, increased **resistance** (narrowing of the system) leads to **decreased flow**, unless the pump produces **increased pressure**. This is described by Poiseuille's Law which states that flow is proportional to pressure drop and the fourth power of the radius of the tube, and is inversely proportional to the length of the tube.

Secondly, during **exercise** resistance in arteries leading to muscle beds decreases, so flow increases **(14a)**. When exercise is undertaken suddenly, CO takes time to catch up so there is an increase in resistance in arteries leading to other systems like the gut **(14c)** (therefore a decrease in flow) to maintain overall BP. Remember, it is a closed system! When CO (HR × SV) is matched to exercise level **(14a)** then flow to gut returns to normal but flow to muscles is increased and BP remains constant throughout. Respiratory rate also increases to clear excess CO_2 **(14a)**.

The diagram below summarizes the factors that regulate peripheral resistance **(14b)**.

↑ resistance ⟶ ↓ flow
unless ♡ ↑ pressure

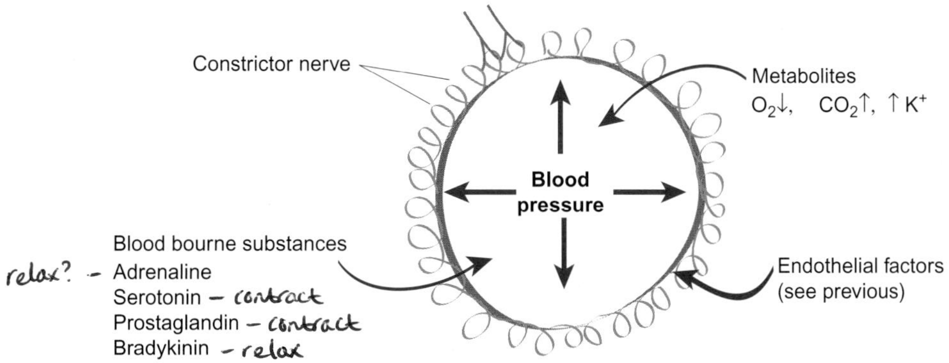

Constrictor nerve

Metabolites
$O_2\downarrow$, $CO_2\uparrow$, $\uparrow K^+$

Blood pressure

Blood bourne substances
relax? – Adrenaline
Serotonin – contract
Prostaglandin – contract
Bradykinin – relax

Endothelial factors
(see previous)

Answers

14. See explanation, d – arterioles
15. A – 3, B – 2, C – 1, D – shortness of breath

16. Regarding the venous system

T **a.** Sixty per cent of total blood volume is in the venous system

f **b.** Upon lying down venous pressure in the limbs increases

T **c.** If a healthy person stands for a long period of time, due to an increase in venous pressure some fluid will leak into the periphery causing oedema

T **d.** Increased pressure in the veins causes a local reflex which increases vascular tone in the arteries

T **e.** Arterial baroreceptors have an important role in autoregulation upon standing

17. Consider the venous system

T **a.** Contraction of lower limb muscles aids venous return to the heart

T **b.** Venous valves prevent retrograde flow

f **c.** During inspiration the intrathoracic pressure increases, which increases venous return

T **d.** During diastole the ventricles relax causing a sucking of venous blood into the heart

f **e.** Veins run in parallel with arteries so pulse pressure can aid venous return to the heart

18. Put the following events into chronological order, regarding the postural reflex

7 **A.** Vasoconstriction occurs in the lower limbs limiting blood flow to the lower limbs

8 **B.** Cardiac output drops

4 **C.** 500 mL of blood is present in the veins of the lower limbs

5 **D.** Baroreceptor reflex causes an increase in heart rate and stroke volume

2 **E.** Healthy individual stands up

6 **F.** A local veno-arterial reflex occurs as a result of vein stretch

1,9 **G.** The difference between arterial and venous pressures is around 90 mmHg

3 **H.** Gravity pulls blood into the lower limbs therefore increasing venous pressure

*BP, blood pressure; HR, heart rate; SV, stroke volume

— 60% of total blood volume

EXPLANATION: THE VENOUS SYSTEM

The longer the tube of blood above the heart, the higher the pressure in the veins and the arteries. Thus when lying down arterial pressure and venous pressure are much the same over the whole body. Upon standing this changes and pressure below the heart increases due to gravity and pressure above the heart decreases (see diagram). But the **difference between the two** (the driving force of blood from the arterial system to the venous system) remains constant (~90 mmHg). This has implications for oedema in heart failure (see page 73). Upon standing, blood pools in the veins of the lower limbs, increasing pressure in the veins and causing stretch. Thus there is less blood in the arterial system and BP drops. This is detected by baroreceptors and atrial receptors and a reflex increase in **HR**, **SV** and **arterial tone** occurs, maintaining BP and increasing venous return to the heart. Venous distension itself causes a local reflex increase in arterial tone. This reduces blood flow to the lower limbs and therefore keeps blood in the thorax.

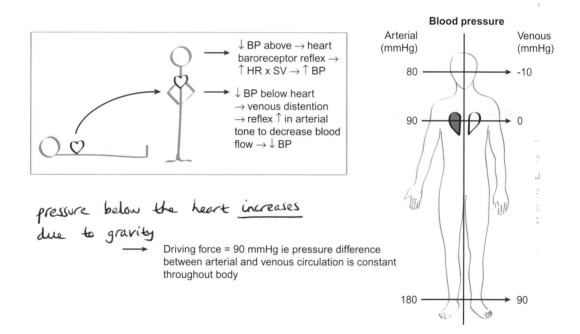

↓ BP above → heart
baroreceptor reflex →
↑ HR x SV → ↑ BP

↓ BP below heart
→ venous distention
→ reflex ↑ in arterial
tone to decrease blood
flow → ↓ BP

Blood pressure

Arterial (mmHg) — Venous (mmHg)

80 → -10

90 → 0

180 → 90

pressure below the heart increases due to gravity

Driving force = 90 mmHg ie pressure difference between arterial and venous circulation is constant throughout body

Venous return is aided by **lower limb muscle contraction, inspiration** (which causes an increase in abdominal pressure, thus increasing the pressure gradient to the heart) and **diastole** of the heart cycle (see page 69).

Answers
16. T F T T T
17. T T F T F
18. 1 – G, 2 – E, 3 – H, 4 – C, 5 – D, 6 – F, 7 – A, 8 – B, 9 – G (point being made: difference ~90 mmHg when standing/lying!)

19. Consider the questions on the microcirculation below. Write brief notes on each

    a. What are the principal components of the microcirculation?
    b. What is the function of the capillaries? What special feature of capillaries allows them to perform this task?
    c. What are the two forces that govern fluid movement in and out of the microcirculation?
    d. Explain what happens in left heart failure which causes fluid in the lungs

20. Answer true or false for each of the following

   f **a.** Hydrostatic pressure is the difference in capillary pressure between the arterial end and the venous end
   T **b.** Hydrostatic pressure drops along the length of the microcirculation from the arterial end to the venous end
   f **c.** Hydrostatic pressure tends to drive fluid into the capillary
   T **d.** A rise in venous pressure causes a rise in hydrostatic pressure
   f **e.** Capillary hydrostatic pressure works in the same direction as osmotic pressure

21. Answer true or false to the following

   T **a.** Albumin and other blood-bound proteins are trapped in the microcirculation
   f **b.** Osmotic pressure is a 'pulling' force driving fluid into the interstitium
   f **c.** Osmotic pressure varies along the length of the microcirculation
   f **d.** Oedema is caused by an increase in blood levels of albumin
   f **e.** In the renal circulation, osmotic pressure is altered to allow fluid filtration into Bowman's capsule

EXPLANATION: THE MICROCIRCULATION

The **microcirculation (19a)** consists of arterioles, capillaries and venules. Capillary walls are only one cell thick and thus allow **diffusion** of important materials in and out of the interstium (oxygen, water, nutrients, hormones, CO_2, creatinine, etc.) **(19b)**.

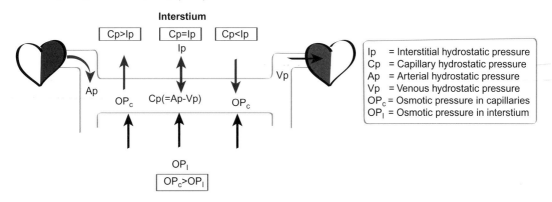

1. HYDROSTATIC   pressure **(19c)** forces fluid out of the capillary and into the interstium. It is the **difference between capillary pressure and pressure in the interstium (Cp − Ip)**. Fluid is filtered out of the compartment with the highest pressure. Since arterial pressure is higher than venous pressure, hydrostatic pressure in the capillary drops from the arterial end to the venous end, therefore filtration and absorption occur (see below).

2. OSMOTIC   pressure **(19c)** is the result of plasma proteins (**colloid osmotic pressure**) and plasma ions (**crystalloid pressure**). Proteins slow down the movement of water molecules, thus the larger the protein content of a compartment the slower the water molecules move and the less likely diffusion is to take place. Unlike ions, which freely diffuse across the capillary wall, proteins are large and are trapped in the capillary, having a constant 'pulling' effect on the fluid in the capillary. Colloid osmotic pressure therefore opposes hydrostatic pressure. The balance of these two forces determines overall fluid filtration. Due to the lower hydrostatic pressure at the venous end, fluid **filtration** may occur here due to colloidal osmotic forces. This relationship is disrupted in heart failure: CP is increased which leads to fluid filtration and pulmonary oedema (see page 75) **(19d)**.

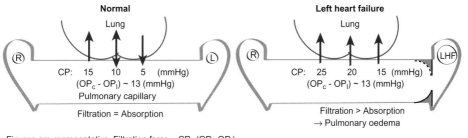

Figures are representative. Filtration force $\approx$ CP -(OP_c-OP_I)

Answers

19. See explanation
20. F T F T F
21. T F F F F

22. Match the options below with the correct volume for a normal sized man

Options

A. 11 L   B. 5.5 L
C. 50 L   D. 35 L
E. 3 L   F. 15 L

1. Total body water   2. Intracellular water
3. Extracellular water   4. Interstitial fluid
5. Blood volume   6. Plasma volume

23. Answer true or false for each of the following:

a. Plasma sodium concentration is normally 145 mmol/L
b. Plasma potassium concentration is greater than intracellular potassium concentration
c. The imbalance of positive ions and negative ions in the plasma is explained by the presence of plasma proteins, which have a negative charge
d. There is normally 22 g/L of albumin in plasma
e. Normal haemoglobin content is around 15 g/dL

24. True or false?

T a. Platelet concentration in the plasma is normally around 250 000/μL
T b. Platelets contain actin and myosin
F c. Platelets are formed in the spleen
F d. A raised neutrophil count is indicative of chronic infection
T e. The red blood cell concentration in the blood is around 5 million/μL

EXPLANATION: FLUID VOLUMES

Unfortunately this all needs to be just memorized. Fluid volumes are calculated as below:

- Total body water (TBW) = 70 per cent of body mass
- Intracellular fluid (ICF) = 70 per cent of TBW
- Extracellular fluid (ECF) = TBW − ICF
- Blood volume = 5.5 L (of which plasma = 3 L)
- Interstitial fluid (ISF) = ECF − plasma volume

	Extracellular fluid	Intracellular fluid	Plasma
$[K^+]$	4.5 mmol/L	140 mmol/L	4 mmol/L
$[Na^+]$	140 mmol/L	10 mmol/L	145 mmol/L
$[Ca^{2+}]$ total	3 mmol/L	1 mmol/L	2.4 mmol/L
$[Ca^{2+}]$ free	1 mmol/L	0.0001 mmol/L	0.96 mmol/L
$[Cl^-]$	110 mmol/L	3 mmol/L	110 mmol/L
$[HCO_3^-]$	24 mmol/L	10 mmol/L	27 mmol/L
Amino acids/protein	10 g/L	120 g/L	70 g/L
pH	7.35	7.0	7.4

Cells found in the blood are as follows:

Cell	Concentration	Function
Erythrocytes	$5 \times 10^6/\mu L$	Carry $O_2 + CO_2$
Total leukocytes	~7000/μL	Defence mechanisms
Lymphocytes	~40%	Cells of chronic infection
Neutrophils	~58%	Cells of acute infection
Monocytes	~2%	Phagocytic cells
Platelets	250 000/μL	Involved in blood clotting

NB White cell numbers and platelet counts vary considerably. This is a rough guide only.

Answers

22. 1 – C, 2 – D, 3 – F, 4 – A, 5 – B, 6 – E
23. T F T F T
24. T T F F T

25. **Answer true or false for each of the following statements:**

T **a.** Haematopoiesis is the formation of red blood cells
T **b.** The liver and spleen are responsible for haematopoiesis for the majority of gestation
T **c.** Red bone marrow in the axial skeleton is the manufacturing site for platelets and RBCs
f **d.** Megakaryocytes (giant cells) repeatedly divide in red bone marrow
f **e.** CFU-E (colony-forming unit for erythrocytes) produces a normoblast which grows into a mature erythrocyte before being released into the bloodstream

26. **Answer the following SAQ regarding haemostasis**

a. What activates the initial response?
b. What chemical messenger released by platelets causes vasoconstriction?
c. Describe how a clot is formed. Details of the intrinsic and extrinsic pathways are not required
d. What factors activate prothrombin?
e. What is measured by the prothrombin time?

27. **Fill in the diagram below with the options listed**

Options

A. Prothrombin   **B.** Thrombin
C. Fibrinogen   **D.** Fibrin monomer

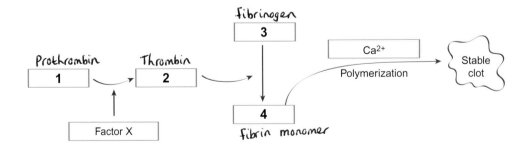

*TXA$_2$, thromboxane A$_2$; ADP, adenosine diphosphate

EXPLANATION: RED BLOOD CELLS

The formation of RBCs and platelets occurs in **red bone marrow** found in the **axial skeleton**, i.e. skull, vertebral column and pelvis. Stem cells in red bone marrow produce colony-forming units (**CFUs**) each colony producing erythrocytes, platelets or neutrophils/monocytes. These cells, called **megakaryocytes**, enlarge through repeated rounds of DNA synthesis **without** cell division. Un-nucleated fragments from these released into the bloodstream form platelets. **Erythrocytes** are formed from normoblasts, the contents of which are internally engulfed leaving only RNA and mitochondria. These then migrate into the bloodstream where they become reticulocytes (following loss of RNA and mitochondria). A day later they mature into erythrocytes. These last for 120 days and are disposed of in the spleen.

Haemostasis in blood vessels is activated when collagen fibres are exposed to the blood **(26a)** (damaged endothelium). Platelets stick to this and activate, releasing **TXA$_2$** which causes vasoconstriction helping to reduce bleeding, and also serotonin and **ADP** which cause activation and aggregation of further platelets to form a platelet plug **(26b)**. This is reinforced by fibrin (discussed below). A strong clot is the result, which then contracts to become tougher and more elastic **(26c)**.

The **intrinsic** and **extrinsic** pathways cause a catalyst reaction forming thrombin from prothrombin **(26d)**. Thrombin then cleaves fibrinogen (soluble) into fibrin monomers (insoluble). In the presence of Ca^{2+} and factor XIII, these form fibrin fibres which then crosslink (thrombin) to strengthen the platelet plug.

Prothrombin time (26e) measures the length of time before coagulation occurs by the route of the extrinsic pathway (via thromboplastin). It takes 14 seconds to complete and is longer if prothrombin or factors V, VII and X are deficient. The intrinsic pathway takes minutes to complete. This is discussed on page 25.

Answers
25. T T T F F
26. See explanation
27. 1 – A, 2 – B, 3 – C, 4 – D

28. **Answer the following regarding hypertension**

    a. Hypertension is a risk factor for a number of diseases. Name four of these
    b. At what blood pressure is hypertension diagnosed? What precautions must one take before making a final diagnosis?
    c. Give a mechanism for the development of primary hypertension
    d. Give two common causes of secondary hypertension
    e. What changes are seen in the walls of the vasculature with long-term hypertension?

29. **Match the class of drug with the most appropriate pharmacological effect. You may use one option more than once or not at all**

Options

    A. Beta-blocker   **B.** Diuretic
    C. Ca^{2+} channel blocker   **D.** ACE inhibitor
    E. Alpha receptor blockers   **F.** Angiotensin II receptor blocker

B **1.** Promotes hypokalaemia by causing an increase in Na^+/K^+ exchange in the nephron of the kidney

A **2.** Has a negative inotropic and chronotropic effect on the heart

A **3.** Causes blockade of beta-1 receptors

C **4.** Inhibits L-type Ca^{2+} entry in smooth and cardiac muscle thus causing vasodilatation and reduction of force generation in the myocardium

B **5.** Increases Na^+ excretion, causing a decrease in blood volume and cardiac output. Blood volume recovers but total peripheral resistance remains decreased

D **6.** Blocks conversion of angiotensin I to angiotensin II

E **7.** Blocks sympathetic activation of vasoconstriction in the periphery, causing vasodilatation

D **8.** Angiotensin II receptor blocker, such as losartan, is a safe alternative to this

D **9.** Also inhibits breakdown of bradykinin, causing a dry cough

*BP, blood pressure

EXPLANATION: HYPERTENSION

Hypertension is a major risk factor **(28a)** for coronary artery disease, heart failure, stroke and renal failure. It is diagnosed at a BP of **140/90 mmHg (28b)** maintained over three separate measurements spanning six months. It may be hereditary and it is also caused by stressful lifestyle, bad diet and lack of exercise.

Essential/primary hypertension (90 per cent) is a multi-factorial problem and a specific cause cannot be found. The probable mechanism involves the kidney as it is this organ that regulates long-term BP. The mechanism is shown below **(28c)**.

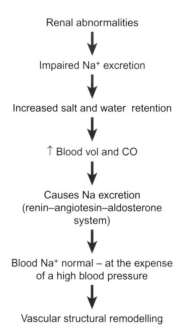

Renal abnormalities

↓

Impaired Na⁺ excretion

↓

Increased salt and water retention

↓

↑ Blood vol and CO

↓

Causes Na excretion
(renin–angiotesin–aldosterone
system)

↓

Blood Na⁺ normal – at the expense
of a high blood pressure

↓

Vascular structural remodelling

In less than 10 per cent the problem is traced to something else (e.g. **hyperthyroidism**, oversecretion of **aldosterone**, or **renal disease**) **(28d)**. Vascular remodelling may occur in muscular arteries – they show progressive thickening of their walls (fibrotic thickening of intima and doubling of internal elastic lamina, plus hypertrophy of muscle layer) **(28e)**.

Beta-blockers, ACE inhibitors, Ca^{2+} channel blockers and diuretics are all first line treatments. These are discussed on page 77 and can be found in the Appendix.

Answers
28. See explanation
29. 1 – B, 2 – A, 3 – A, 4 – C, 5 – B, 6 – D, 7 – E, 8 – D, 9 – D

30. Clinical case study

A young couple in their mid-twenties are brought into the Emergency Department. Forty minutes ago they were involved in a motor traffic accident. The man, who was in the passenger seat, is unconscious and is receiving immediate medical attention from your superiors. You speak to the woman who is concerned for her partner, anxious and confused. She is feeling faint, and looks pale. After a quick examination her BP is 110/90 mmHg and her pulse is 104 bpm. You tell her to sit down and you get a cup of tea for her.

Half an hour later you return bearing tea (you got distracted by another patient) to find the woman unconscious.

- **a.** What do you think has caused her unconsciousness?
- **b.** What aspects of her apparently innocent arrival into the Emergency Department are in hindsight suspicious?
- **c.** What other tests would you have liked to perform in hindsight?
- **d.** What is your next step?

Investigation shows that she has ruptured her spleen and is bleeding internally. She is taken to theatre.

- **e.** Give an account of the physiological mechanisms that have maintained her blood pressure

You feel guilty as you feel you should have noticed and acted sooner.

- **f.** Would her haemoglobin have been altered had you done a blood test?
- **g.** What will determine if this woman lives or dies, assuming surgery to correct the internal bleeding is successful? What is the mechanism behind irreversible shock?

---

*BP, blood pressure; HR, heart rate; CO, cardiac output

EXPLANATION: SHOCK

Shock is defined as **circulatory failure** resulting in inadequate organ perfusion. This could be due to pump failure (heart failure, see page 73) or circulatory failure.

In this case the woman has a concealed haemorrhage, and is losing circulating volume. The early warning signs are tachycardia, confusion, anxiety, postural hypotension, pallor and sweating. BP may appear normal with only a reduction of pulse pressure being apparent. A lying and standing BP should be taken to determine if the patient is hypovolaemic. Haemoglobin levels would appear normal as the blood loss is acute so the body has no time to mobilize fluid from other compartments (which would then lower the haemoglobin concentration). The emergency treatment is to get intravenous access and give her fluids or blood, plus oxygen and get her to theatre.

Young people cope with this situation particularly well, BP being maintained with up to 30 per cent blood volume gone (see graph below). The acute drop in blood flow is detected by baroreceptors and peripheral and central chemoreceptors which activate vasoconstriction in veins and arteries and increase the HR. Blood flow to the heart and brain remains the same but supply to other organs (e.g. gut and skin) are reduced. The kidney begins water retention (thus urine output is low) but this takes more time. These are marked on the graph as 'reflexes'.

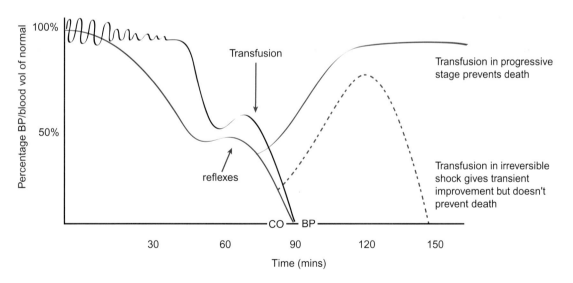

Irreversible shock occurs due to lack of oxygen and toxicity to the tissues causing multi-organ failure. If a transfusion is given at this stage a transient recovery in BP is seen but leads to the eventual death of the patient. The transfusion needs to occur before this tissue damage takes place – the 'Golden Hour'.

Answers

30. See explanation

31. Regarding clotting disorders

a. Name two disorders of clotting
b. Anticoagulation therapy is often prescribed after operations. Give two reasons for this
c. What is the problem with anticoagulation therapy?

32. Match the mechanism of action with the drugs listed below. You may use the same option more than once or not at all

Options

A. Heparin

B. Warfarin

C. Streptokinase

D. Aspirin

E. Factor VIII

F. Factor X

D **1.** Inhibits platelet thromboxane A_2 synthesis, thus reducing platelet activation and aggregation during clot formation

B **2.** Takes 2 days to have an effect

B **3.** Vitamin K analogue

C **4.** Lyses thrombi by activation of plasminogen to plasmin

A **5.** Increases rate of antithrombin III–thrombin complex formation, inactivating thrombin

B **6.** Modifies factors VII, XI, X and prothrombin

A **7.** Short acting

*DVT, deep vein thrombosis; PE, pulmonary embolism; AF, atrial fibrillation; MI, myocardial infarction; PLD, phospholipase D

EXPLANATION: CLOTTING AND ANTICOAGULATION

One important disorder of clotting is **haemophilia (31a)**. This is a genetic defect in which factor VIII or factor IX is absent. A more common major cause of bleeding is **anticoagulation therapy (31b)**. Anticoagulation is given to people with the following:

- Recurrent DVT
- Past/recurrent PE
- Prosthetic heart valve
- AF.

Thrombi are a disorder of clotting which can occur due to blood stasis (DVT, AF) or abnormal endothelium (MI, stroke) – both cause infarction. Anticoagulation therapy is often prescribed after operations as the patient may be immobilized for a long period of time during recovery. Immobilization increases the risk of DVT and subsequent PE (similarly to long flights) **(31b)**. Warfarin interacts with a lot of drugs and getting the levels right for the desired level of anticoagulation (i.e. to reduce thrombus formation) is tricky. If levels become too high then bleeding can occur **(31c)**.

Here is a diagram of the intrinsic and extrinsic pathways of clot formation showing how the drugs mentioned in question 32 exert their effect.

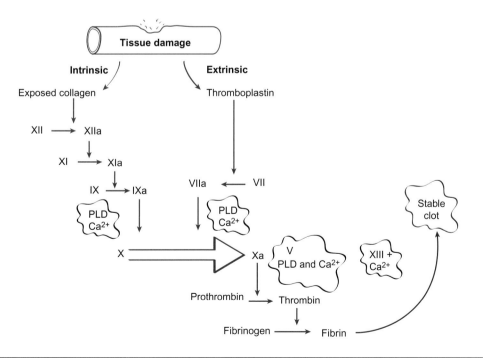

Answers

31. See explanation
32. 1 – D, 2 – B, 3 – B, 4 – C, 5 – A, 6 – B, 7 – A

33. Case study

A 35-year-old Australian woman comes into the Emergency Department. She flew into England last night after a 24-hour flight, and woke up this morning with a slight fever. She noticed that her right leg was red, swollen and warm. She has been on the contraceptive pill for the last year.

a. What is the likely diagnosis?

b. What is causing the swelling and the pain?

While waiting in the Emergency Department to be sent up to the ward, she developed severe breathlessness and fainted. When she came around she complained of palpitations and stabbing pain when breathing in. Her jugular veinous pressure (JVP) was raised, her BP was low, and she was centrally cyanosed.

c. What complication has occurred?

d. What investigations would you perform to confirm your hypothesis?

e. What treatment would you suggest?

f. Is this condition life threatening? Explain your answer

---

*DVT, deep vein thrombosis; VF, ventricular fibrillation; CT, computed tomography; ECG, electrocardiogram; PE, pulmonary embolism

EXPLANATION: DEEP VEIN THROMBOSIS

Embolism formation is a complication of blood stasis, or hypercoagulability. This can result from prolonged bed rest (commonly after surgery) or, as in this case, a long flight. In addition, conditions such as thrombophilia and pregnancy (some consider it a condition!), and drugs such as the oral contraceptive pill and hormone replacement therapy (HRT) confer extra risk.

The likely cause of her swollen leg is a DVT, associated with low grade pyrexia. Another (unlikely) cause of one swollen leg is cellulitis. Two swollen legs suggest a systemic disease such as right heart failure. It is highly unlikely that DVTs will occur in both legs.

A thrombus has blocked a vein (commonly below the knee) and thus the route that the blood takes back to the heart is blocked. This causes pooling of blood behind the clot (like a traffic jam due to a car accident). This leads to inflammation – hence the pyrexia and warmth of the leg.

A complication of DVT is a **pulmonary embolism**. A section of the thrombus may break off and travel through the right side of the heart and get lodged in the pulmonary system. If a major artery is blocked this can lead to death very quickly. It presents with syncope, pleuritic chest pain and palpitations. Central cyanosis occurs because the blood cannot get past the clot to get to the alveolar membranes and thus is not oxygenated. Underperfusion of the heart may lead to VF and death.

A chest X-ray would probably reveal little so a CT scan is needed. An ECG may also show some abnormality.

High flow oxygen is needed immediately. Anticoagulation should also be started (heparin), with **warfarin** treatment following for three months afterwards.

Answers

33. See explanation

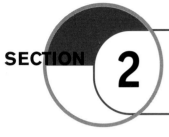

BLOOD SUPPLY TO THE HEART

1. Concerning the coronary arteries. True or false?

T **a.** The left coronary artery gives rise to the circumflex artery and anterior interventricular artery/left anterior descending artery

F **b.** The atrioventricular (AV) node is supplied by the AV nodal artery which arises from the left coronary artery

T **c.** Both left and right coronary arteries supply the sinoatrial node

T **d.** The right coronary artery gives off the right marginal and posterior interventricular arteries

F **e.** The left ventricle is supplied by the circumflex artery and the right marginal artery

2. Regarding the coronary arteries

T **a.** The right ventricle and apex are supplied by the marginal artery

T **b.** The interventricular septum and both ventricles are supplied by the posterior interventricular artery arising from the right coronary

F **c.** There are no anastomoses between the anterior interventricular artery and the posterior interventricular artery

F **d.** Having a greater number of collateral arteries is a disadvantage during cardiac ischaemia

T **e.** A thrombus in the anterior interventricular artery has a poorer prognosis than a thrombus in the marginal artery

3. Regarding venous and nervous distribution in the heart

F **a.** The great cardiac vein joins with the left marginal, left posterior ventricular, small and middle cardiac veins to drain into the superior vena cava

T **b.** The heart's nervous supply comes from autonomic nerve fibres from the cardiac plexus

T **c.** The cervical and superior thoracic parts of the sympathetic trunks give rise to the heart's sympathetic innervation

F **d.** Parasympathetic innervation arises from the IX cranial nerve (glossopharyngeal)

F **e.** Stimulation of the sympathetic fibres causes the sinoatrial node and atrioventricular node to slow the heart rate down so more oxygen can be supplied to the myocardium

---

*CO, cardiac output; MI, myocardial infarction; SA node, sinoatrial node; AV node, atrioventricular node

EXPLANATION: ANATOMY OF THE CORONARY ARTERIES

The coronary arteries are distributed as shown below.

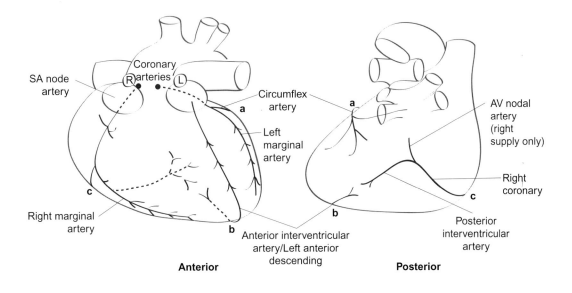

Anterior   **Posterior**

The first arteries given off by the aorta are not the brachiocephalic trunk as commonly thought, but in fact the **right** and **left coronary arteries**, originating in the right and left coronary sinuses superior to the right and left cusps of the aortic valve respectively. The distribution is shown above. The most important artery supplies the left ventricle (which is responsible for CO) and is called the **anterior interventricular artery** (or if you are a surgeon, the left anterior descending). An MI involving this artery is not good as CO is severely diminished, resulting in rapid cardiac failure. Anastomoses between branches of the left and right coronary are widespread and are useful. During an MI, collateral arteries open up and may supply blood to the area of infarction in a retrograde manner, therefore saving the myocardium from necrosis.

The SA node receives its blood supply from both the right coronary artery (60 per cent) and the left coronary artery (40 per cent). If one is occluded, then local vasodilatation in the patent artery can supply sufficient blood for function to be maintained. The AV node is only supplied by the right coronary.

Answers

1. T F T T F
2. T T F F T
3. F T T F F

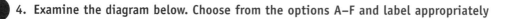

4. Examine the diagram below. Choose from the options A–F and label appropriately

Options

A. Anterior interventricular artery
B. Right marginal artery
C. Circumflex branch
D. Right coronary artery
E. Left coronary artery
F. Left marginal artery

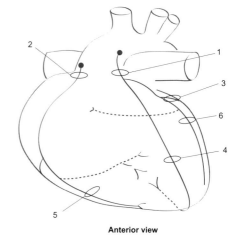

Anterior view

5. Examine the diagram and label it from the options below

Options

A. Great cardiac vein
B. Left marginal vein
C. Coronary sinus
D. Middle cardiac vein
E. Left posterior cardiac vein
F. Venae cordis minimae

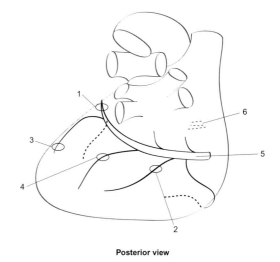

Posterior view

*SA node, sinoatrial node; AV node, atrioventricular node; HR, heart rate

EXPLANATION: VEINS AND NERVES OF THE HEART

The anatomy of the coronary arteries is discussed on the previous page so you should have answered question 4 correctly!

The venous distribution is relatively simple. The heart is drained in two ways: first by small veins that empty straight into the right atrium (**venae cordis minimae** and **anterior cardiac veins**) and secondly, and more importantly, by veins that empty in to the **coronary sinus** and again into the **right atrium**. The coronary sinus runs from left to right across the atrioventricular groove on the posterior surface of the heart. It receives the great cardiac vein, middle and small cardiac veins as it travels from left to right. In addition the left posterior and marginal veins also open up into the coronary sinus.

The anatomy of the nervous system supplying the heart is also straightforward. The heart is supplied by **auto-nomic nerve fibres** derived from the cardiac plexus, which is sandwiched between the bifurcation of the trachea and the arch of the aorta (see page 49). The **sympathetic supply** comes from cervical and upper thoracic parts of the sympathetic trunks, whereas the **parasympathetic supply** is derived from the vagus nerve (see page 85). The post-ganglionic fibres end in the SA node and AV node and modify impulse generation, muscle contractility and coronary blood flow. Sympathetic stimulation increases all of the above, resulting in faster HR, increased force of contraction and vasodilatation of the coronary arteries. Parasympathetic stimulus has the opposite effect (but does not affect contractility).

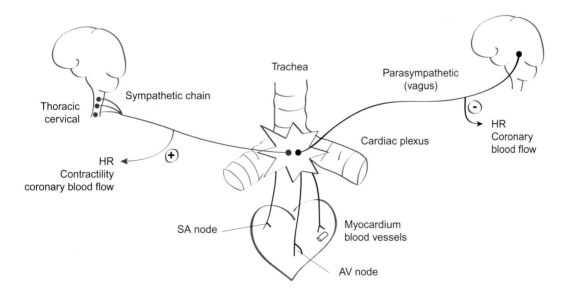

6. With regard to the flow of blood through the coronary arteries, answer true or false

F **a.** The flow is described as 'phasic' as there is higher flow in the left coronary artery when the heart is in systole

T **b.** The right coronary flow is greatest during diastole

T **c.** At a heart rate of 70 beats per minute, left coronary blood flow can be as much as 300 mL/min

T **d.** Left coronary flow is greater than right coronary flow

T **e.** As the heart rate increases, blood flow to the myocardium increases

7. With regard to coronary flow

T **a.** As heart rate increases systolic time decreases

T **b.** During exercise coronary flow can increase up to four-fold

F **c.** Coronary flow is controlled via the cardiac plexus only

T **d.** The myocardium has a high capillary density, with one capillary for every myocyte

T **e.** High capillary density allows the myocardium to extract a high proportion (70 per cent) of available oxygen from the blood

8. With regard to flow through the coronary arteries

a. It is increased due to sympathetic stimulation from the cardiac plexus

b. It is increased when oxygen demand increases

c. It is increased as hypokalaemia develops

d. Adenosine has no impact on coronary flow

e. Glyceryl trinitrate (GTN) spray is given to people suffering from angina and works by vasodilation of the coronary arteries to relieve ischaemic pain

*HR, heart rate

EXPLANATION: CORONARY BLOOD FLOW

Coronary blood flow is described as **phasic**. This is because it varies throughout the duration of the cardiac cycle. The flow through the left coronary artery decreases during systole, as pressures produced by the left side of the heart exceeds pressure in the artery and compressive forces reduce blood flow. Therefore 85 per cent of blood flow to the left side of the heart occurs during diastole. Conversely, the right side of the heart does not produce the same magnitude of pressure, so right coronary flow increases during systole as the pressure in the aorta increases (i.e. as blood is pumped out of the heart).

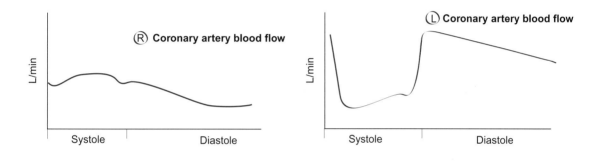

During exercise or tachycardia the HR increases, and the diastolic interval is therefore reduced, allowing less time for left coronary blood flow. This is compensated by the action of **hypoxia**, **hyperkalaemia** and **adenosine**, which cause coronary vasodilatation and thus increase blood flow four-fold. In elderly persons, vasodilatation is impaired and this leads to ischaemic pain (when oxygen demand is not met) on exertion.

Answers

6. F T T T T
7. T T F T T
8. T T F F T

9. Regarding the circulation

a. Put the following organs in order, starting with the system that receives most blood flow and ending with the least **at rest**
   A. Heart
   B. Brain
   C. Kidney
   D. Muscle
   E. Skin
b. Which metabolites are responsible for an increase in the brain's blood flow?
c. Cerebral flow is regulated between the pressure limits of 60 and 140 mmHg. What implications does this have for blood flow to the brain?
d. **(i)** Draw a simple graph to represent phasic flow through the coronary vessels. Label the systolic and diastolic components
   (ii) How is blood flow to the myocardium affected during exercise?
   (iii) Name two methods of increasing blood flow to the myocardium
e. What percentage of total blood flow supplies the kidneys? Name three chemical or hormonal factors that affect this supply

*CO, cardiac output; NO, nitric oxide; AngII, angiotensin II

EXPLANATION: THE CIRCULATION

The three most important circulations to understand are those of the brain, heart and kidneys. The others vary greatly depending on the state of exercise. The kidney receives 22 per cent of the blood supply, muscle 15 per cent, the brain 14 per cent, skin 6 per cent and the heart 4 per cent at rest (NB 1 per cent = 50 mL/min, therefore the heart receives 200 mL/min, for example).

1. BRAIN. Blood flow is kept constant **(9c)** (at 700 mL/min or 15 per cent of CO) within the limits stated in question 9(c) and is regulated by **autoregulation** and the concentration of metabolites. CO_2 and H^+ **(9b)** cause cerebral depression so must be disposed of – hence an increase in blood flow. An increase in O_2 levels will cause a decrease in blood flow. Sympathetic nervous control also causes vasoconstriction in arteries leading to the brain to prevent an increase in intracranial pressure.

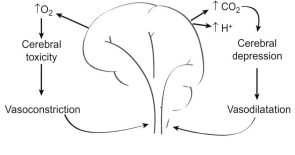

2. HEART. The myocardium extracts **70 per cent** of oxygen from the coronary blood supply, which is a higher proportion than in other organs. However, when the myocardium requires more oxygen, adenosine and K^+ are released, causing vasodilatation (see page 35).

3. RENAL. The blood supply to the kidneys is very high (**1200 mL/min or 22 per cent of CO**) **(9e)**. Blood flow stays constant for arterial pressures between 80 and 170 mmHg so the **glomerular filtration rate** (GFR) is always maintained. The hormonal control is summarized in the diagram below.

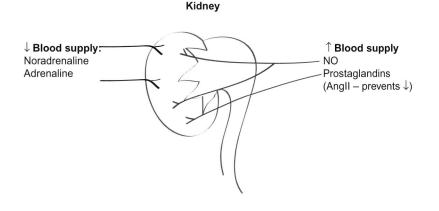

Kidney

10. Case study

A 62-year-old man visits his GP. He is a long-term smoker who has hypertension. Recently, he has been suffering from retrosternal discomfort and describes the pain as heaviness on the front of his chest. Sometimes it radiates to his neck and jaw. Precipitating factors include walking up stairs to his bedroom and being shouted at by his wife. He needs to rest for 5 minutes before the pain disappears. He sometimes feels out of breath as well.

    a. Give two possible diagnoses that would account for his symptoms

    b. What is causing his pain?

The GP referred his patient to a cardiologist. Blood tests and ECGs were done and the only finding of note was a lowered haemoglobin of 10.2 g/dL. There was no abnormality on ECG and thyroid function was normal.

    c. Could the anaemia be responsible for his chest pain? What is the mechanism?

The patient was sent for an exercise tolerance test which showed reduced exercise tolerance and lowered ST segment on the ECG.

    d. What is the likely diagnosis?

The man's condition was explained to him, and treatment discussed.

    e. What would your advice be to the patient?

    f. What medication would you suggest?

Two years later, the man's symptoms were found to have increased and the medication was ineffective.

    g. Are there any further investigations that need to be performed? What are the treatment options now?

---

*ECG, electrocardiogram; HR, heart rate; MI, myocardial infarction

EXPLANATION: ANGINA CASE STUDY

This is an extremely common complaint in western society. Changes in lifestyle have meant increased incidence of coronary artery disease and atherosclerosis and a corresponding increase in **angina**.

The angina pain described by the patient is a **retrosternal crushing pain** radiating to the **neck**, **face** and **left arm**. It is due to myocardial ischaemia as the blood supply to the myocardium on exertion is increased. As the heart rate increases, diastolic time and therefore blood supply to the myocardium decreases. In healthy individuals this is dealt with by drastic vasodilatation of the coronary artery. However, in cases like this one the coronary artery is furred up and is unable to dilate during exertion. Therefore the ischaemia causes pain.

The pain is similar during an angina attack and an MI. However angina pain is **reversible on rest and medication**. A resting ECG is normally unremarkable.

Anaemia is also a cause of chest pain, as the blood's oxygen carrying ability is decreased and therefore ischaemia occurs via a different mechanism. These two often go together.

An exercise ECG raises the heart rate and causes ischaemic pain. The ECG may show **ST segment depression** consistent with myocardial ischaemia, which then disappears upon resting.

The first advice to this patient would be to stop smoking and to look at ways to lose weight. Treatment to deal with issues such as hypertension and anaemia would be next on the list. Medical treatment includes **aspirin**, which reduces mortality, a **beta-blocker** to reduce heart rate, **nitrate spray** to reduce symptoms when needed, and a **Ca^{2+} antagonist** to reduce total peripheral resistance (TPR) so the heart has less work to do, reducing the contractility of the myocardium and therefore reducing oxygen demand. Iron supplements should be given.

Two years on, an angiogram should be performed to assess extent of the disease and **angioplasty** or **coronary artery bypass operation** should be considered.

Answers

10. See explanation

11. Consider the pathology of angina and answer true or false to the following

a. Ischaemic pain is due to stenosis of the coronary artery which prevents increased blood supply reaching the myocardium in times of increased demand
b. Coronary vessel narrowing is due to atherosclerosis in the majority of cases
c. Concentric atheromatous plaques are plaques affecting one side of the coronary artery, and blood flow can be improved by drug therapy
d. Atherosclerosis is due to macrophage infiltration into the intima and release of high density lipoprotein (HDL)
e. The disease is reversible

12. Which of the following are risk factors for developing angina secondary to atherosclerosis?

a. Inherited factors
b. Female gender
c. Old age
d. Diabetes mellitus
e. Obesity
f. Hyperlipidaemia
g. Smoking
h. Low blood pressure
i. Japanese race

13. Match the pathophysiological descriptions 1–4 with the types of angina listed below

Options

A. Stable angina
B. Unstable angina
C. Variant angina
D. Decubitus angina

1. Predictable angina that occurs during exercise and stress resulting from increased demand of oxygen by the myocardium which cannot be satisfied by the blood supply
2. Chest pain at rest caused by an increase in coronary artery vascular tone. Attacks are worse in the morning. Mechanism unknown
3. Unpredictable pain not related to exercise. Chest pain increases with frequency and intensity. Due to variable luminal stenosis. Associated with a greatly increased chance of myocardial infarction
4. Chest pain upon lying flat

---

*HDL, high density lipoprotein; LDL, low density lipoprotein; MI, myocardial infarction; BP, blood pressure; Mφ, macrophage

EXPLANATION: TYPES OF ANGINA

Stable angina is the most common form of angina. It is due to **atherosclerosis** of the coronary arteries. The process is shown in the diagram below, with progression labelled 1–6.

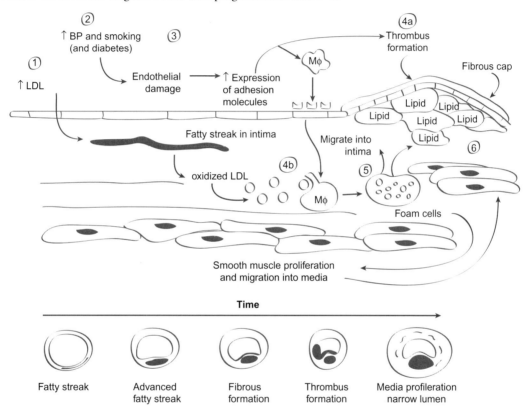

Factors that predispose to atherosclerosis are familial traits, being male (2:1 under 55), being white, being old, having hypertension or diabetes, having high cholesterol, smoking and eating a high fat diet.

It is thought that the atherosclerosis process is started by damage to the endothelium, which allows LDL to migrate into the intima. Damage may be caused by long-term smoking or hypertension. Diabetes causes damage to the endothelium, making atherosclerosis almost inevitable.

Unstable angina is due to reversible ischaemia caused by variable luminal stenosis of some segments of the coronary arteries. **Variant angina** is a result of vasospasm as a result of increased vascular tone. Attacks are self-limiting and rarely lead to MI. **Decubitus angina** is very rare.

Answers
11. T T F F F
12. T F T T T T T F F
13. 1 –A, 2 – C, 3 – B, 4 – D

14. Case study

You are the house officer on duty and it has been a long night. You are just considering the possibility of getting a coffee to prevent collapse when a 58-year-old man is brought into the Emergency Department. The complaint is of severe central crushing chest pain extending into the left arm and shortness of breath. The pain had started suddenly when he was having breakfast and had become unbearable over the last 3 hours at work. Nitrate spray is ineffective. Nothing relieved the pain.

    a. What is the suspected diagnosis?

    b. How do you manage at this stage?

Upon further questioning you discover that his father died from a heart attack at 65. He has previously suffered from angina.

    c. Are these factors relevant? Are there any other factors that you would like to know about his past medical history?

Upon examination he is tachycardic, tachypnoeic, and has a BP of 150/95 mmHg. His JVP is raised. Bi-basal crackles can be heard in the lungs.

    d. What is the significance of the bi-basal crackles? What could be responsible for this?

Bloods come back showing an increased erythrocyte sedimentation rate (ESR), increased levels of creatine kinase and a positive troponin T test.

    e. Discuss the blood test results. Do they support your original diagnosis?

---

*BP, blood pressure; JVP, jugular venous pressure; MI, myocardial infarction; COPD, chronic obstructive pulmonary disease; tPA, tissue plasminogen activators; Trop T, troponin T; CK, creatine kinase; LDH, lactate dehydrogenase

EXPLANATION: MYOCARDIAL INFARCTION

This is an **MI**, the result of a coronary artery becoming occluded after an atheromatous plaque ruptures. Platelet activation and thrombosis occurs in the lumen of the coronary artery, leading to complete occlusion. The myocardium distal to the occlusion receives no blood and the pain is a result of ischaemia and necrosis of this tissue. **Time is muscle** in this situation and the sooner flow is restored to the ischaemic tissue, the better the long-term prognosis.

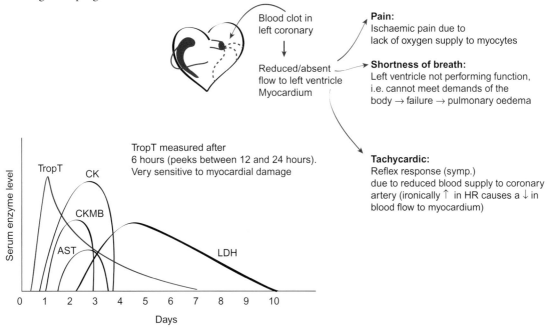

Blood clot in left coronary

↓

Reduced/absent flow to left ventricle Myocardium

Pain:
Ischaemic pain due to lack of oxygen supply to myocytes

Shortness of breath:
Left ventricle not performing function, i.e. cannot meet demands of the body → failure → pulmonary oedema

Tachycardic:
Reflex response (symp.) due to reduced blood supply to coronary artery (ironically ↑ in HR causes a ↓ in blood flow to myocardium)

TropT measured after 6 hours (peeks between 12 and 24 hours). Very sensitive to myocardial damage

Risk factors for MI are similar to those for angina discussed previously. Anything that predisposes to atheromatous change leads to a chance of developing MI. Smoking, high cholesterol, hypertension and family history of MI are the most important to consider.

Assuming this is an MI, **aspirin** is given immediately. **Oxygen** to aid breathing and **morphine** to relieve pain and anxiety is also administered. These should be prescribed with care and contraindications, such as liver disease or COPD, fully considered. **Streptokinase** or **tPA** ('clot-busters') should also be given immediately, assuming there are no contraindications. The longer that you wait, the more myocardium is destroyed and the poorer the prognosis.

The symptoms are explained in the diagram above. Blood tests for cardiac enzymes also give valuable information. These leak out of ischaemic myocytes into the blood.

Answers

14. See explanation

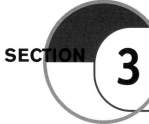

THE HEART

3 THE HEART

1. Consider the developing heart in the fetus. Answer true or false

a. At day 18 the heart is located in the same position you would expect an adult heart to be found
b. The heart is derived from the mesoderm of the embryo
c. The right and left ventricles pump blood in parallel
d. The primitive heart consists of five chambers
e. The primitive heart is formed at week 23

2. In the developing heart

a. Septation is the formation of the atrial septum
b. Around 40 per cent of the cardiac output is diverted from the right side of the heart to the left
c. Foramen ovale is a persistent hole left in the ventricular septum to divert blood
d. Ligamentum arteriosum is a bypass mechanism in the fetus which diverts blood from the pulmonary artery to the aorta
e. Oxygenation of blood occurs as fetal blood passes through the placenta

3. Fill in the paragraph below using the following options

Options

A. Placenta	B. Foramen ovale
C. Pulmonary system	D. Ligamentum arteriosum
E. Right ventricle	F. 24 weeks
G. Left atrium	H. Ductus arteriosus
I. Aorta	J. Birth

In the fetus oxygenation of blood occurs in the **1**, as the lungs are undeveloped and receive no oxygen. As a result, no blood is sent through the **2**. Blood entering the right atrium is shunted through the **3** into the **4**. Some blood enters the right ventricle and passes into the pulmonary trunk. This blood is shunted again by the **5**, which joins the pulmonary trunk with the **6**. This is seen as the **7** in adults. These shunts are closed at **8**.

EXPLANATION: THE FETAL HEART

At day 18 the fetus consists of a **primitive streak**, and three layers: the **endoderm**, the **mesoderm** and the **ecto-derm**. The ectoderm forms the skin and nervous system, the mesoderm forms the 'insides' and the endoderm is destined to be the gut lining. At this stage the heart, composed of mesoderm, is in two pieces on the left and right. Complex foldings bring these together to form one primitive heart tube consisting of six chambers. More complex foldings later and the heart is recognizable as an adult's.

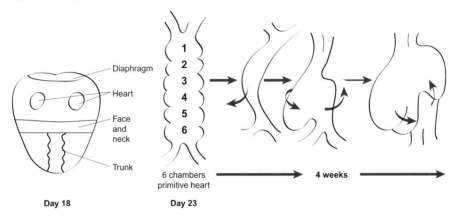

The primitive atrium is destined to become two. A **septum primum** develops and forms the **foramen primum** which closes up once the septum is completed by growth. A second hole, the **foramen secondum** is formed. A second septum then grows and part of the first septum degenerates. The result is the **foramen ovale**, which acts as a right to left shunt. The **ductus arteriosus** is also a right to left shunt and joins the pulmonary trunk with the aorta.

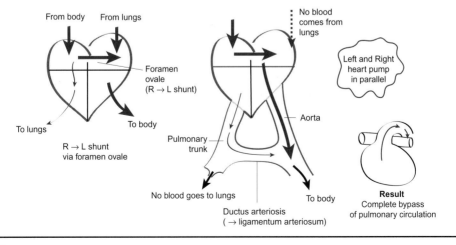

Answers
1. F T T F F
2. T F F T T
3. 1 – A, 2 – C, 3 – B, 4 – G, 5 – H, 6 – I, 7 – D, 8 – J

4. Consider the gross anatomy of the heart and answer true or false

    a. The heart lies in the anterior mediastinum
    b. The bifurcation of the trachea is posterior to the heart
    c. The heart lies posterior to the body of the sternum and the second to the sixth costal cartilages at the level of T5–T8 vertebrae
    d. The apex of the heart can be found on the left in the fifth intercostal space along the mid-axillary line
    e. The right ventricle lies upon the left hemi-diaphragm

5. Regarding the gross anatomy of the heart

    a. The arch of the aorta is found at the sternal angle at the level of T4
    b. The pulmonary trunk is anterior to the ascending aorta
    c. The superior vena cava is anterior to the pulmonary trunk and posterior to the ascending aorta
    d. The descending aorta travels posteriorly to the oesophagus
    e. The superior vena cava drains straight into the left atrium

6. Consider the gross anatomy of the heart

    a. The ascending aorta is 2.5 cm in diameter
    b. The arch of the aorta gives rise to the brachiocephalic trunk which becomes the left common carotid and left subclavian arteries
    c. During systole, blood flows from the atria to the respective ventricles
    d. Oxygenated blood is pumped out of both ventricles to their destination via either the pulmonary trunk or the aorta
    e. The heart is normally larger than half the width of the entire mediastinum

*SVC, superior vena cava; LCC, left common carotid; RCC, right common carotid; LSA, left subclavian artery; RSA, right subclavian artery

EXPLANATION: ANATOMY OF THE MEDIASTINUM (i)

The anatomy of the mediastinum is described over the next two pages, as it is important that you are familiar with it. There are four parts:

- **Superior mediastinum** contains left lobe of thymus, arch of aorta, oesophagus, trachea (U-shaped costal cartilages) and SVC
- **Middle mediastinum** contains the heart and both lung roots
- **Posterior mediastinum** contains thoracic duct, azygos vein, hemizygous veins, aorta and oesophagus
- **Anterior mediastinum**.

An important landmark is the **sternal angle**, at the spinal level **T4**. Starting from most anterior, going posteriorly, you see the ascending aorta and the arch of the aorta travelling posteriorly, the SVC, the pulmonary trunk and bifurcation, the trachea birfurcation and then the oesophagus. The course of the ascending arch and then descending aorta should be noted in relation to the other structures.

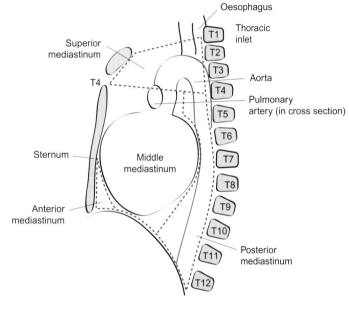

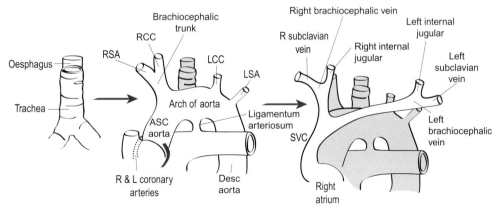

The branches of the aorta are shown above. The first arteries to come off the aorta are the left and right coronary arteries. The **brachiocephalic trunk** which becomes the **right common carotid** and **right subclavian** is next. The **left common carotid** and **left subclavian** come off the arch of the aorta as individual arteries.

7. Examine the radiograph below and supply the labels from the following options

Options

A. Clavicle   B. Left hilum
C. Superior vena cava   D. Right ventricle
E. Left ventricle   F. Aortic knuckle
G. Right atrium   H. Left hemi-diaphragm

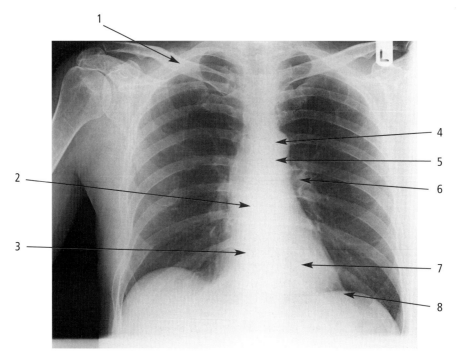

Courtesy of Professor Michael Marber and Dr Matthew Faircloth.

EXPLANATION: ANATOMY OF THE MEDIASTINUM (ii)

The chest radiograph is also important and will be first line examination in any cardiology or respiratory case. A diagram representing what can be seen on a well exposed radiograph is shown below. Normally both lung fields are clear and the left and right heart borders are clearly visible. The costo-diaphragmatic angles are sharp and the pulmonary arteries can also be seen. The heart is less than half the width of the entire mediastinum. Any enlargement of the heart greater than this is pathological. In cardiac problems pulmonary oedema is seen as a clouding of the lung fields and is representative of left ventricular inability to cope with demand.

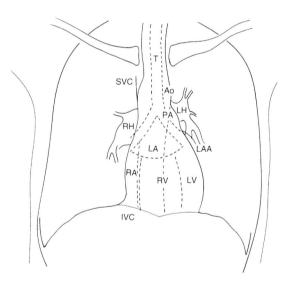

Ao	Aortic Knuckle
SVC	Superior Vena Cava
PA	Main trunk of the pulmonary artery
RH	Right hilum
LH	Left hilum
LA	Left atrium
LAA	Position of left atrial appendage
RA	Right atrium
RV	Right ventricle
LV	Left ventricle
IVC	Position of inferior vena cava

From Roberts, G.M., Hughes, J.P., Hourihan, M.D., *Clinical Radiology for Medical Students*, Butterworth Heinemann, 1998.

Answers

7. 1 – A, 2 – G, 3 – D, 4 – F, 5 – C, 6 – B, 7 – E, 8 – H

8. Consider the anatomy of the pericardium

    a. The pericardium is a double-walled fibrous sac that encloses the heart
    b. The pericardium is fused with the central tendon of the diaphragm
    c. The fibrous pericardium protects the heart from trauma
    d. The parietal pericardium forms the epicardium of the heart
    e. The visceral pericardium is reflected off the great vessels and is continuous with the parietal pericardium

9. Regarding the anatomy of the pericardium

    a. Fluid in the potential space between the parietal and visceral layers of the pericardium is pathological
    b. Arterial supply of the pericardium is derived partially from the internal thoracic artery
    c. Coronary arteries supply the visceral layer of the pericardium
    d. The phrenic nerve, roots C3–C6, supplies the pericardium
    e. Cranial nerve X (the vagus nerve) supplies the pericardium

10. Consider the anatomy of the heart

    a. The most superficial layer of the heart is the endocardium
    b. The myocardium is composed of cardiac muscle
    c. The blood supply for the myocardium is derived from the coronary arteries
    d. Cardiac muscle is histologically identical to smooth muscle
    e. Sensory supply of the myocardium is via the sympathetic trunk of the upper four thoracic nerves

EXPLANATION: THE PERICARDIUM

The outermost layer seen upon opening the chest is the **fibrous pericardium**. This is inelastic and protects the heart against sudden overfilling. It is connected to the diaphragm, the posterior surface of the sternum and the tunica adventitia of the great vessels. Next is the **parietal layer** which is reflected off the heart and great vessels and becomes the **visceral layer** intimately related to the myocardium. Between these two layers (the pericardial cavity) is a thin film of fluid which allows the heart to move freely within the sac without friction or irritation. The visceral pericardium comprises the outermost layer of the heart, the epicardium. The myocardium, which contains cardiac muscle, is below that and the endocardium is the internal lining of the heart.

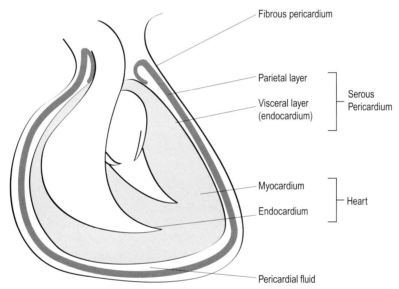

Supply of the pericardium is from the **phrenic nerve** 'C3, 4, 5 keeps you alive!', the tenth cranial nerve (**the vagus**) and the **sympathetic trunk**. Sensory afferents from the myocardium enter the sympathetic trunk via the posterior roots of the upper four thoracic nerves. Thus ischaemic cardiac pain is 'referred' to the areas of skin supplied by the upper four thoracic nerves. This is why the pain is sometimes felt in the shoulder and neck.

Answers
8. T T F F T
9. F T T F T
10. F T T F T

11. True or false? In the anatomy of the heart

a. The inferior and superior vena cavae open up into the right atrium
b. The coronary sinus drains into the right atrium
c. The right atrium makes up the right border of the heart
d. Muscular pectinati are found in the right atrium
e. The atrioventricular septum has the fossa ovalis, a remnant of the foramen ovale

12. Consider the right ventricle

a. The right ventricle forms the sternocostal surface and makes up the inferior border of the heart
b. The right ventricle myocardium is three times as thick as the left ventricle myocardium
c. The outflow tract of the right ventricle is the pulmonary vein, carrying venous blood to be oxygenated by the lungs
d. The right ventricle contracts before the left ventricle during the cardiac cycle
e. The blood supply of the right ventricle consists of the right marginal branch of the right coronary artery

13. Consider the anatomy of the heart

a. The left atrium forms the base of the heart
b. The left atrium contains deoxygenated blood
c. Two pulmonary veins enter the posterior wall
d. The left atrium and the right atrium contract together during systole
e. The left auricle can be seen on a chest X-ray

14. Consider the anatomy of the heart

a. The left ventricle forms the diaphragmatic surface of the heart
b. The left ventricle is seen as the left border of the heart in a chest X-ray
c. The left ventricle receives oxygenated blood from the lungs via the left atrium
d. The left ventricle produces more pressure than the right ventricle
e. The outflow tract is via the arch of the aorta

---

*SVC, superior vena cava; RA, right atrium; IVC, inferior vena cava; RV, right ventricle; LV, left ventricle

EXPLANATION: ANATOMY OF THE HEART

The anatomy of the heart is best learnt in diagrammatic form.

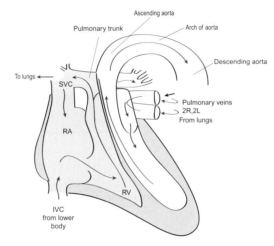

The route the blood takes during the cardiac cycle (discussed on page 69) is important. Deoxygenated blood enters the RA via the IVC, SVC and coronary sinus. It then moves into the RV which, during systole, pumps the blood to the lungs via the pulmonary trunk and subsequently right and left pulmonary arteries. Oxygenated blood returns to the left atrium from the lungs via four (two superior, two inferior) pulmonary veins. This blood moves into the LV and is then subsequently pumped into the ascending aorta. The LV is twice as thick as the right as it has to produce much more pressure. Both atria and both ventricles contract together (diastole and systole respectively).

The atria both consist of a smooth internal lining, and a more muscular (rough) lining called musculi pectinati. The fossa ovalis is found in the atrial septum (see page 47) which is the remains of the foramen ovale. Anatomy of the heart is a large subject and cannot be addressed here in detail, however it is important!

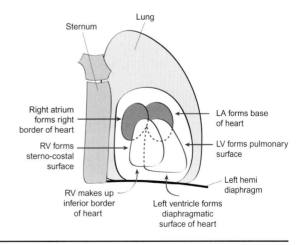

The route the blood takes during the cardiac cycle (discussed on page 69) ... The fossa ovalis is found in the atrial septum (see page 47)

Answers
11. T T T T F
12. T F F F T
13. T F F F T
14. T T T T F

15. Match the correct valve given below with the following statements. You may use the same option more than once and you do not have to use all options

Options

A. Mitral valve

C. Aortic valve

E. Tricuspid valve

B. Bicuspid valve

D. Pulmonary valve

1. This valve leads from the right atrium to the right ventricle
2. This valve is composed of three cusps
3. This valve has two papillary muscles connected to the endocardium
4. This valve is most frequently diseased
5. This valve consists of three **semilunar** cusps and is found at the level of the third intercostal cartilage
6. This valve consists of three **semilunar** cusps and is found at the level of the third intercostal space
7. Found just superior to the right and left cusps of this valve is the opening of the right and left coronary arteries

16. Consider the diagrams below and answer the following questions

    a. Which valves are represented by these two diagrams?
    b. Label parts 1–6 with the options provided below:

Options

A. Right semilunar cusp

B. Left coronary artery

C. Papillary muscle

D. Semilunar cusp

E. Chordae tendineae

F. Valve cusp

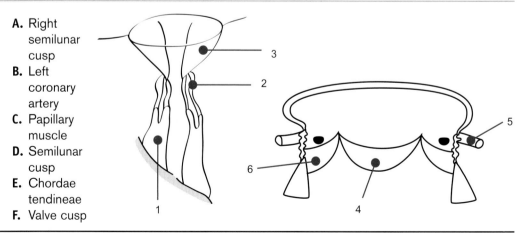

EXPLANATION: THE VALVES

There are essentially only two types of heart valve: the ones that guard the atrioventricular orifices and the ones that guard the outflow tracts.

The **tricuspid** and **mitral** (or bicuspid) valves guard the right and left atrioventricular orifices respectively. These consist of **valve cusps**, attached to which are **chordae tendineae**, which attach to the **papillary muscles** of the endocardium. In the same way as an operator flying a kite at constant altitude pulls on the kite string to stop the kite flying away, the papillary muscles pull on the chordae tendineae to stop the cusps flailing into the atrium during systole. When the direction of blood is from the atrium to the ventricle the valves offer no resistence to flow (only the pressure in the ventricle does – see page 69), but during systole, when pressure in the ventricle far exceeds pressure in the atrium, the valve slams shut, fully closing off the atrioventricular orifice, so the blood may flow out of the heart via the ouflow tracts. The tricuspid valve has three cusps as its name suggests and the mitral valve has two cusps and corresponding chordae tendineae and papillary muscles.

The aortic and pulmonary valves are identical and need no extra machinery to work. They consist of three **semilunar cusps** which open during systole when pressure in the ventricles exceeds the pressure in the outflow tracts, and slam shut when flow starts to reverse. The only difference is that the right and left coronary arteries are given off just above the right and left cusps of the aortic valve respectively.

For surface anatomy, see page 71.

Answers

15. 1 – E, 2 – E, 3 – A, 4 – A, 5 – D, 6 – C, 7 – C
16a. Left – mitral, right – aortic
16b. 1 – C, 2 – E, 3 – F, 4 – D, 5 – B, 6 – A

17. Consider the histology of the heart and answer true or false

   a. The myocardium consists of skeletal muscle cells called myocytes
   b. Myocytes have a much less organized appearance than smooth muscle
   c. Myocytes are rich in mitochondria
   d. Intercalated discs allow the myocardium to act as a 'functional syncytium'
   e. Gap junctions made up of connexons confer structural stability to adjacent myocytes

18. Consider the histology of the heart

   a. Myocytes contain both actin and myosin
   b. A, H and I bands are classically seen in the microstructure of the myocardium
   c. Z lines represent myosin bands
   d. Sarcoplasmic reticulum is more extensive in cardiac muscle than in skeletal muscle
   e. A terminal cisternal sarcoplasmic reticulum and a t-tubule form a diad

19. Consider the histology of smooth muscle

   a. Smooth muscle is found in blood vessels, airways and the gastrointestinal tract
   b. Smooth muscle does not contain actin filaments
   c. Myosin fibres are aligned into sarcomeres
   d. Dense bodies are seen under microscopy and these are drawn together during contraction
   e. Smooth muscle cells are joined to the extracellular matrix by integrins

*SR, sarcoplasmic reticulum; ATP, adenosine triphosphate

EXPLANATION: HISTOLOGY OF THE HEART

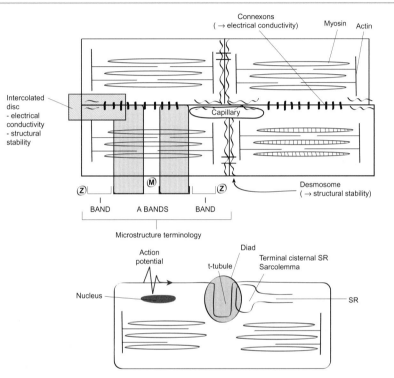

The microstructure of a cardiac myocyte is shown above. The structure is somewhere in between smooth muscle and skeletal muscle. The myocardium acts as a functional **syncytium** thanks to the intercalated discs. Gap junctions made up of **connexons** confer electrical conductivity, which is vital in impulse spread through the myocardium, and **desmosomes** add structural stability. The cell membrane of a myocyte (called the sarcolemma) receives the action potential from neighbouring myocytes. The sarcolemma infolds every now and again to form a t-tubule and meets the terminal cisternal SR at the end of the SR, which is vital in muscle contraction. Ca^{2+} released from the SR binds to troponin C and activates the binding between myosin and actin (using ATP). Actin and myosin are aligned into sarcomeres, which are effectively units of power; the tension produced by all elements is summated in a particular direction.

Smooth muscle is less organized than cardiac muscle but has the same components. The cells are larger in size but contain less volume than myocytes. Actin and myosin pull on intermediate fibres attached to the inner surface of the cell membrane via dense bodies. The cell membrane is attached to the extracellular matrix by integrins thus allowing manipulation of the external environment.

The full mechanism of contraction is discussed on pages 61 and 63.

Answers
17. F F T T F
18. T T F F T
19. T F F T T

20. With regard to cardiac muscle, is it true or false that

a. Ca^{2+} is responsible for the plateau of the action potential
b. Calsequestrin binds to Ca^{2+} in the sarcoplasmic reticulum
c. Ca^{2+} stored in the SR is released into the cytoplasm when the action potential activates a voltage-operated Ca^{2+} channel
d. Muscle contraction force can be regulated by altering either Ca^{2+} entrance into cytoplasm or Ca^{2+} storage
e. The concentration of Ca^{2+} reaches a peak level of about 2 M

21. With regard to cardiac muscle

a. When Ca^{2+} concentration rises above 100 nM the majority of the intracellular Ca^{2+} is pumped out of the cytoplasm back into the extracellular space
b. The Na^+/Ca^{2+} exchanger in the sarcolemma pumps excess Ca^{2+} out of the cell
c. Digoxin (a positive inotrope) increases contractility by indirectly acting against Ca^{2+} removal from the cell
d. An increase in heart rate automatically causes a decrease in contractility
e. Negative inotropes are used in the treatment of heart failure

22. Put these events in the correct chronological order

A. Ca^{2+} is pumped back into the tubular sarcoplasmic reticulum via adenosine triphosphate pumps
B. Crossbridge cycle occurs
C. During the plateau phase of the action potential, voltage-operated Ca^{2+} channels in the sarcolemma are activated
D. Ca^{2+} activates Ca^{2+} release from in the tubular sarcoplasmic reticulum
E. Ca^{2+} is pumped out of the cell via Na^+/Ca^{2+} exchanger using a Na^+ gradient created by the Na^+/K^+ ATPase
F. The action potential travels down the sarcolemma of the myocyte
G. A rapid influx of Ca^{2+} occurs over the next 10 ms
H. A small amount of extracellular Ca^{2+} enters the cytoplasm

---

*VOCC, voltage-operated Ca^{2+} channel; SR, sarcoplasmic reticulum; HR, heart rate; ATP, adenosine triphosphate

EXPLANATION: THE MECHANISMS OF CONTRACTION

All types of muscle use Ca^{2+} to bring about contraction, but in different ways.

In cardiac muscle Ca^{2+} enters the cell via VOCCs in the **sarcolemma t-tubules**. This small rise in Ca^{2+} induces further release from the **tubular SR**. The final levels of Ca^{2+} in the cell depend on how fast the myocyte is contracting. If the HR is fast, the myocyte does not have enough time to recover fully. Therefore less Ca^{2+} can be pumped out of the cell ready for the next contraction so intracellular levels rise. This has implications in the control of heart failure. When levels reach 100 nM, Ca^{2+} is pumped back into the SR by Ca^{2+} ATPases and outside the cell by Na^+/Ca^{2+} exchangers (the Na^+ gradient maintained by the Na^+/K^+ exchanger). Peak levels of Ca^{2+} can reach 2 µM (remember that Ca^{2+} channels are slow to react).

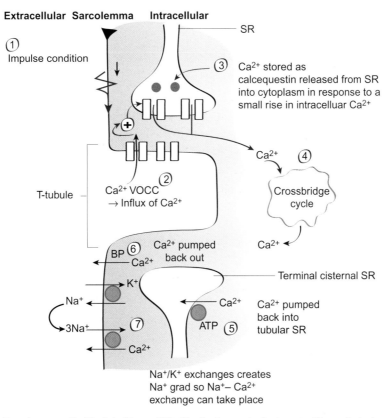

From Aaronson, Pl., Ward, J., Wiener, C.M., *The Cardiovascular System at a Glance*, 2nd edn, 2003. Redrawn with kind permission of Blackwell Science Ltd.

Answers
20. T T F T F
21. F T T F T
22. 1 – F, 2 – C, 3 – H, 4 – D, 5 – G, 6 – B, 7 – A, 8 – E

23. **Fit the following options into boxes 1–5 in the diagram below**

Options

A. Calmodulin
C. Myosin light chain kinase
E. Dephosphorylated myosin

B. Crossbridge cycle
D. Phosphorylated myosin

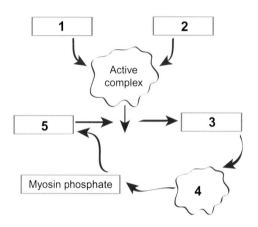

24. **Put the descriptions below into either of the two groups. You may use each option more than once or not at all**

Options

A. Ca^{2+} triggers contraction
C. Shortens more
E. ATP consumption higher

B. Contains troponin
D. Crossbridge cycle slower
F. No fatigue

Group 1: Smooth muscle
Group 2: Skeletal muscle

---

*ADP, adenosine diphosphate; cAMP, cyclic adenosine monophosphate; IP3, inositol-(1,4,5)-trisphosphate; SR, sarcoplasmic reticulum

EXPLANATION: SMOOTH MUSCLE

Smooth muscle is found in blood vessels and therefore has a bearing on blood pressure control. Upon membrane excitation by chemical/pharmacological stimulus, free Ca^{2+} ions are released from storage in the SR, via the secondary messenger IP_3, and bind to **calmodulin** (a Ca^{2+} binding protein). This complex activates **myosin light chain kinase** which phosphorylates the myosin chain and permits it to bind to actin. The cross-bridge cycle follows (force generation step). ADP dissociates and myosin is subsequently dephosphorylated.

Cardiac and skeletal muscle contraction is controlled differently. In skeletal muscle, the troponin complex regulates access to the myosin binding site on actin. Troponin C binds to Ca^{2+} and this causes a conformational change, allowing myosin access to its binding site on actin.

Drug control of cardiac muscle and smooth muscle has implications for management of heart failure and high blood pressure (see pages 21, 77 and appendix). For example, digoxin inhibits the Na^+ pump, thereby increasing $[Na^+]$ in the cytosol. This has the effect of decreasing the gradient that drives the Na^+/Ca^{2+} exchanger and therefore less Ca^{2+} is removed from the cell (see page 61). Because there is more Ca^{2+} in the cell, greater tension is produced by the cell and this acts as a positive inotrope. During exercise, less time is available for pumping Ca^{2+} out of the cell before the next cycle begins (because the heart is beating at a faster rate) and thus more tension is produced. Another positive inotrope, noradrenaline from sympathetic nerve fibres, increases cAMP levels, resulting in increased Ca^{2+} entry into the cell causing an increase in contractility. Remember that positive inotropes are contra-indicated for long term treatment of heart failure as the increased tension produced by the myocytes accelerates the condition and increases mortality.

Ca^{2+} channel blockers are used for the control of blood pressure because they stop Ca^{2+} entering the cell and therefore reduce contraction, lowering blood pressure. This is discussed more on page 77.

Answers
23. 1 – A, 2 – C, 3 – D, 4 – B, 5 – E
24. Group 1 – A, C, D, F; Group 2 – A, B, E

25. A 70-kg man has a heart rate of 70 bpm, an end diastolic volume of 120 mL and an end systolic volume of 50 mL.

    a. What is his CO?
    b. What three general factors influence cardiac output?
    c. What must occur in the heart for an increase in cardiac output?
    d. On the axis provided below, draw the relationship between end diastolic pressure and stroke volume
    e. How is this explained at the molecular level?

SV

EDP

26. True or false? End diastolic volume is

    a. Independent of end diastolic pressure
    b. Dependent on compliance
    c. Dependent on sympathetic tone
    d. Unaffected in heart failure
    e. Increased in the right ventricle if central venous pressure increases

27. Consider Starling's Law

    a. It states that the work generated by the myocyte is increased proportionately with increased fibre length
    b. As the fibre length increases, more crossbridges can be formed between actin and myosin, up to a point
    d. As fibre length increases, troponin becomes less sensitive to Ca^{2+}
    e. Stroke volumes of the left and right ventricles are matched as a consequence of Starling's Law
    f. When heart rate and contractility are constant, central venous pressure determines cardiac output

---

*EDV, end diastolic volume; ESV, end systolic volume; CO, cardiac output; SV, stroke volume; HR, heart rate; EDP, end diastolic pressure; LV, left ventricle; CVP, central venous pressure

EXPLANATION: CARDIAC OUTPUT (i) – CONTRACTILITY AND STARLING'S LAW

The three factors that influence CO are preload (venous pressure), afterload (arterial pressure) and cardiac status (contractility and rate) **(25b)**. An immensely important formula to remember is **CO = SV × HR (25a)**. It follows that CO can be controlled by modifying either SV or HR.

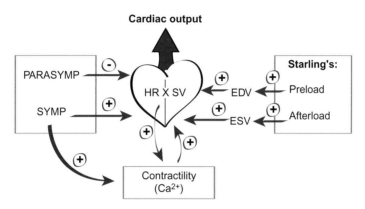

1. If **preload** is increased (CVP) then EDP and thus EDV increase (blowing harder into the balloon for a fixed period of time means more air in the balloon). This depends on the compliance (how easy the balloon is to inflate) of the heart. An increase in EDV causes an increase in stretch of the myocardium (or balloon!) due to the increased volume of blood, which results in an increase in contraction force (Starling's Law, see page 67).

2. If **afterload** is increased (blood pressure) then pumping against this increased pressure is harder for the heart. Less blood is pumped out of the LV, which results in an increased end systolic pressure and ESV, which again results in ventricular stretch during diastole (increased EDV) and the next contraction will produce more force (Starling's Law), thereby restoring cardiac output.

3. **HR** is modified by sympathetic and parasympathetic stimulation. As HR increases there is less time for Ca^{2+} to be removed from the myocytes, and thus more Ca^{2+} is retained. This results in an increase in peak Ca^{2+} concentration during systole, and force increases. This is referred to as an increase in **contractility**, i.e. more force for the *same fibre length*. Noradrenaline (sympathetic stimulation) also increases contractility by increasing Ca^{2+} entry into the myocyte. An increase in EDP does not increase contractility, though it increases force (cf. Starling's Law) **(25c,e)**.

Answers

25. a = (120–50) × 70; b,c,e see explanation; d see Q29
26. F T T F T
27. F T F T T

28. The following factors alter contractility (true or false?)

a. An increase in heart rate
b. Noradrenaline acting on beta-receptors
c. Change in pH
d. Digoxin
e. End diastolic pressure

29. SAQ: Consider the graph below

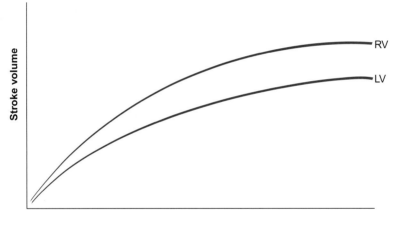

End diastolic pressure

a. Using evidence from the graph, why is the end diastolic pressure higher in the left ventricle than in the right?
b. Draw on the graph the left ventricular function curve of a failing heart. Why does this cause problems?
c. How is a normal cardiac output maintained during heart failure?

EXPLANATION: CARDIAC OUTPUT (ii) – CONTRACTILITY AND STARLING'S LAW

First let us clarify the definition of **contractility**. It is a change in force generation **not** due to a change in fibre length (EDP) and thus nothing to do with Starling's Law. It **is** a change in force generation due to an increase in HR, noradrenaline or digoxin (which all increase Ca^{2+} entry into the cell and thus increase force generation). Therefore an increase in HR that does not allow enough time for Ca^{2+} to be pumped out of the cell, sympathetic stimulation and digoxin all increase contractility. **EDP** does **not** alter **contractility** but affects muscle fibre length in the myocyte.

In contrast, **Starling's Law** states that the energy released during contraction depends on the initial fibre length. This is based on the **sliding filament theory**. As length increases due to an increase in EDV (see page 65), more crossbridges are formed (reduced overlap of the actin filament so more force may be generated). Once fibre length increases past 2.25 μm (optimum) the actin filaments leave a gap and so less crossbridges can be formed. In cardiac muscle there is also a length-dependent increase in Ca^{2+} sensitivity of **troponin C**, which is believed to play a vital role.

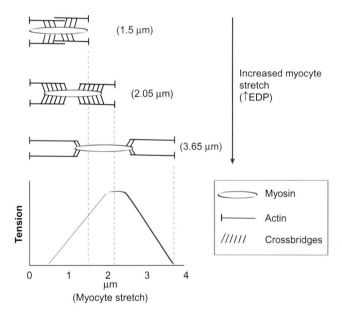

As a result of Starling's Law, SV of the right and left ventricles are matched **(29a)**, but due to the difference in compliance the LV operates at a higher EDP than the right. In left heart failure the ventricular function curve is depressed and CO is maintained at the expense of an increased EDP at rest **(29c)**. Therefore any increase in SV that is needed upon exertion cannot be met by the ventricle.

Answers

28. T T T T F
29. See explanation. For b, see page 75

30. Put the following statements in the correct chronological order

Options

A. Contraction of the atria completes ventricular filling
B. Aortic and pulmonary valves shut
C. The end diastolic volume is 120 mL
D. Atrial pressure rises until atrioventricular valves open
E. The C-wave occurs because isovolumetric contraction of the ventricles causes the mitral/tricuspid valves to bulge into the atria
F. Aortic and pulmonary valves open and blood is ejected into outflow tracts
G. Dicrotic notch occurs during a brief reversal of flow
H. Venous blood pressure (5 mmHg) is responsible for some filling of the ventricles
I. The ventricles relax
J. The ventricles contract and the tricuspid valve closes

31. Consider the graph below demonstrating the pressure changes seen throughout the length of one cardiac cycle

a. Fill in the boxes provided with the following options

Options

A. MO (mitral valve opens)   **B.** MC (mitral valve closes)
C. AO (aortic valve opens)   **D.** AC (aortic valve closes)

b. Indicate the duration of one cycle if the HR is 60 pbm. Which section of the cardiac cycle shortens significantly during exercise?

c. State normal values for end diastolic and end systolic volumes. Use this to work out the stroke volume from your figures

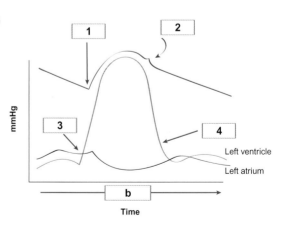

From Aaronson, Pl., Ward, J., Wiener, C.M., *The Cardiovascular System at a Glance*, second edition, 2003. Redrawn with kind permission of Blackwell Science Ltd.

*MV, mitral valve; EDP, end diastolic pressure; AV, aortic valve; EDV, end diastolic volume; LV, left ventricle; ESV, end systolic volume; SV, stroke volume

EXPLANATION: THE CARDIAC CYCLE (i)

1. ATRIAL SYSTOLE.   This facilitates the movement of venous blood from both atria into the respective ventricles. At rest, however, it accounts for only 20 per cent of ventricular filling, the other 80 per cent resulting from venous pressure. The importance of the atria for filling increases as heart rate rises and in exercise.

STATUS:		MV (and tricuspid valve) OPEN	End Diastolic Pressure = 10mmHg

2. ISOVOLUMETRIC CONTRACTION.   This simply means that the ventricles contract but the volume of blood in them does not change. Therefore the pressure increases sharply (imagine standing on a balloon). For this to happen both inlet and the outlet tracts must be closed.

STATUS:		MV and AV CLOSED	End Diastolic Vol = 120 mL of blood

3. EJECTION.   Just like your balloon, when the pressure becomes too great the contents escape by the easiest route possible, and volume decreases. In the case of the heart, the route is the outflow tract via the AV. Once the pressure in the LV exceeds that of the aorta, the AV is forced open and blood is forced out of the ventricle. This will continue as long as pressure in the ventricle is greater than in the outflow tract. As the pressures equalize, flow becomes less and eventually, when pressure in the aorta is higher than in the ventricle, the AV slams shut again to prevent backflow into the ventricle (seen as dicrotic notch on pressure trace).

STATUS:		AV OPEN (and MV closed)	End Systolic Vol = 50 mL Stroke Vol = 70 mL

This is continued on page 71.

Answers

30. 1 – H, 2 – A, 3 – C, 4 – J, 5 – E, 6 – F, 7 – G, 8 – B, 9 – I, 10 – D
31a. 1 – C, 2 – D, 3 – B, 4 – A
31b. 1 sec, diastole
31c. SV = EDV–ESV = 70 mL

32. State true or false for each of the following

a. Venous filling pressure is around 15 mmHg
b. At rest venous filling pressure is responsible for 80 per cent of ventricular filling
c. The a-wave on the pressure trace represents contraction of the ventricles
d. The end diastolic volume is 120 mL
e. The end diastolic pressure is 40 mmHg

33. State true or false for each of the following

a. Isovolumetric contraction of the left ventricle occurs when both the mitral and aortic valve are shut
b. The pressure in the aorta during the isovolumetric contraction phase is less than in the ventricle
c. The C-wave represents bulging of the mitral/tricuspid valve into the atrium
d. When pressure in the left ventricle exceeds 80 mmHg (pressure in the aorta) the aortic valve opens
e. The dicrotic notch occurs when the aortic valve opens

34. With regards to the heart sounds heard on auscultation, assign options A–F to the statements below

Options

A. Mid diastolic murmur
C. S1
E. Early diastolic murmur

B. Ejection systolic murmur
D. Pansystolic murmur
F. S2

1. The atrioventricular valves closing
2. This sound is a low frequency 'lubb'
3. The aortic and pulmonary valves closing
4. Mitral stenosis
5. Mitral regurgitation
6. Aortic stenosis
7. Aortic regurgitation

*MV, mitral valve; AV, aortic valve; LV, left ventricle; SV, stroke volume; EDP, end diastolic pressure; JVP, jugular venous pressure

EXPLANATION: THE CARDIAC CYCLE (ii)

4. DIASTOLE.   The ventricles relax and expand and the pressure drops rapidly. Once this pressure is lower than the pressure in the atria then the MV opens and ventricular filling commences. This is split into two stages: one rapid, where the expanding ventricle 'sucks' blood in, and the second where the ventricle is fully relaxed and filling is due to venous pressure alone.

STATUS:	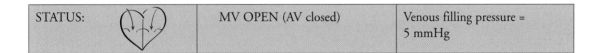	MV OPEN (AV closed)	Venous filling pressure = 5 mmHg

Pressure changes throughout the cardiac cycle may be visualized by pulsations in the neck (JVP). The a-wave of this pressure trace is seen as the atria contract. The v-wave is seen as the ventricles contract. The c-wave is a pressure increase in the atrium due to the mitral/tricuspid bulge during isovolumetric contraction.

This is one complete cardiac cycle. The efficiency of the cardiac cycle depends on the correct functioning of the valves. The way to work out flow is to imagine the pressures involved. Blood only flows from one compartment to another because the pressure in the first is larger than in the second. Therefore the aortic valve will only open once the pressure in the ventricle exceeds (diastolic) pressure in the aorta. The valves are there to prevent backflow. Once the pressure in the aorta is greater than the LV the AV is shut.

Auscultation areas are shown in the diagram below. PAMT (pulmonary, aortic, mitral, tricuspid) lie anatomically in a relatively straight line. Auscultation areas, however, are the final destination of the blood flowing through the valves, e.g. blood flowing through the MV ends up at the apex. Murmurs are dealt with further on page 79.

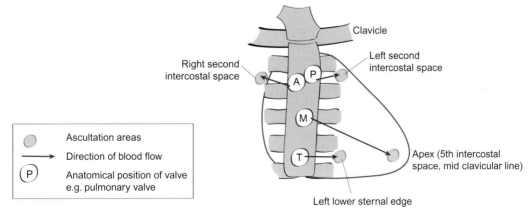

Answers
32. F T F T F
33. T F T T F
34. 1 – C, 2 – C, 3 – F, 4 – A, 5 – D, 6 – B, 7 – E

35. The following can cause heart failure (true or false?)

a. Ischaemic heart disease
b. Cardiomyopathies
c. Valvular disease
d. Cirrhosis of the liver
e. Pregnancy

36. The following may occur during heart failure

a. Inability to provide adequate cardiac output to maintain tissue needs during exertion
b. Increased left venticular contractility
c. Increased left ventricular compliance
d. Hypertrophy of left ventricular myocardium
e. Pulmonary oedema

37. Which of the following options occur in (1) left heart failure, (2) right heart failure? You may use an option more than once or not at all

Options

A. Dyspnoea
B. Pleural effusions
C. Pitting ankle oedema
D. Raised jugular venous pressure
E. Atrial fibrillation
F. Hepatomegaly
G. Orthopnoea
H. Chest pain

38. As part of compensation during heart failure the neurohumoral system is activated. Put these events in the correct chronological order

A. Na$^+$ and water retention
B. Blood pressure returns to normal
C. Activation of the renin-angiotensin system
D. Decreased cardiac output and low blood pressure
E. Increase in cardiac output and vasoconstriction in renal arteries
F. Increased central venous pressure and end diastolic pressure
G. Increased sympathetic stimulation

*CO, cardiac output; EDP, end diastolic pressure; LV, left ventricle; RV, right ventricle; CVP, central venous pressure

EXPLANATION: HEART FAILURE – PHYSIOLOGY

Heart failure is a broad term used to describe an **inadequate CO** needed to support the needs of the tissues, or can only do so at the expense of a raised EDP.

The causes are numerous. The main categories are: **heart muscle disease** (e.g. ischaemic heart disease), **restricted filling** (e.g. pericarditis), **inadequate heart rate**, **excessive preload** (e.g. mitral regurgitation or fluid overload) and **chronic excess afterload** (e.g. aortic stenosis, hypertension).

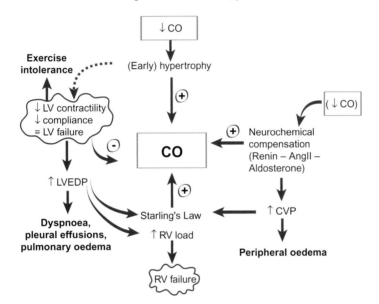

From Aaronson, PI., Ward, J., Wiener, C.M., *The Cardiovascular System at a Glance*, 2nd edn, 2003. Redrawn with kind permission of Blackwell Science Ltd.

The diagram above shows the compensatory mechanisms during heart failure. These seem like a good idea at the time (i.e. maintaining CO) but unfortunately they cause progression of heart failure and eventually the patient becomes decompensated. Increased sympathetic tone long term and renin-angiotensin system activation cause Ca^{2+} overloading in myocytes. This reduces the effectiveness of the Ca^{2+} channels, causes mitochondrial damage and decreased compliance, reducing the effectiveness of the myocardium as a result.

Hypertrophy causes an increase in muscle cell size due to more intracellular contractile elements. In addition, extracellular collagen deposition occurs and together these reduce compliance and contractility. Hypertrophy also causes valve defects by enlarging the atrioventricular passage so the valve is no longer large enough to cover it completely (regurgitation) and decreases coronary capillary density of the myocardium, resulting in ischaemic pain. Past MI may leave scar tissue and further reduce the pumping efficiency of the ventricle.

Answers
35. T T T F T
36. T F F T T
37. 1 – A, B, G, E, H; 2 – C, D, E, F
38. 1 – D, 2 – G, 3 – E, 4 – C, 5 – A, 6 – B, 7 – F

39. A 72-year-old man is brought into the Emergency Department. Over the past few days he has experienced recurrent chest pains and dyspnoea, made worse by lying flat (orthopnoea). A chest radiograph is performed and shown below

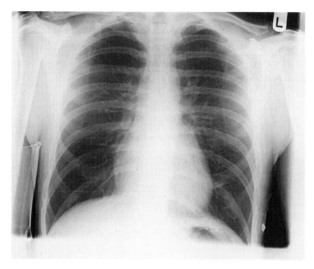

Courtesy of Professor Michael Marber and Dr Matthew Faircloth.

a. Name five risk factors for heart disease
b. Does this man have an enlarged heart? What features of the radiograph are abnormal?
c. Explain why there is bi-basal shadowing in the lung fields. What would you expect to hear upon auscultation of the lung bases?

An echocardiogram demonstrates an ejection fraction of 35 per cent with akinesia of the septum and apex of the left ventricle. Upon referral to a cardiologist a pansystolic murmur is appreciated at the apex that radiates to the axilla. Heart rate is 140 bpm and blood pressure is low.

d. What is the normal ejection fraction? What does the akinesia of the left ventricle suggest about this man's past medical history?
e. What is the significance of the murmur heard? Is this a contributory factor to the man's problems?
f. What is a possible reason for his chest pain? Would drug therapy to slow the heart rate down help? Name a drug that is used
g. What additional drug therapy if any would you suggest? Are there any other interventions you would consider?

---

*MI, myocardial infarction; EDP, end diastolic pressure; LV, left ventricle; CO, cardiac output; SV, stroke volume; HR, heart rate; LHF, left heart failure

EXPLANATION: HEART FAILURE – CLINICAL ASPECTS

The mechanisms described on page 73 make the ventricle less efficient and start to fail as a pump, which results in increased EDP. This increased pressure is transmitted backwards through the system. In LV failure the pressure backs up into the left atrium and pulmonary system. This increases the hydrostatic pressure in the pulmonary vessels causing net movement of fluid out of the capillary and into lung interstium resulting in **shortness of breath** (explained on page 15). The same mechanism occurs in right heart failure, except that the pressure is backed into the systemic venous circulation, and therefore fluid moves out of capillaries into the periphery (**ankle oedema, ascities and hepatomegaly**).

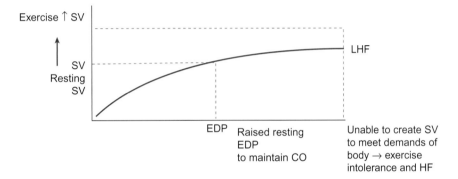

Exercise intolerance is due to resting effort. In a person with heart failure the heart and body are working flat out to maintain resting CO. Any effort that requires an increase in CO will result in **exertional dyspnoea** as the EDP rises in the LV in an attempt to increase SV, thus causing pulmonary oedema. **Exertional angina** is also experienced due to low cardiac output and, as the HR increases to improve CO (reflex) coronary blood flow is decreased further (due to ↓ diastolic time).

Clinically, heart failure presents with exertional dyspnoea and chest discomfort. A chest radiograph may show **cardiomegaly** (>50 per cent cardiothoracic ratio), prominent upper lobe veins, lung field shadowing due to peripheral oedema (gravity dependent) and possibly pleural effusions. Echocardiography is the investigation of choice and may show valve dysfunction (see page 79) or ventricle dysfunction (ejection fraction below 60 per cent is abnormal) and may show akinesia of a portion of the myocardium demonstrating a previous MI (scar tissue).

Answers
39. See explanation

40. Match the drug actions below with the correct class of drug. You may use the same answers more than once or not at all

Options

    A. ACE inhibitors
    B. Angiotensin receptor antagonist
    C. Cardiac glycosides
    D. Loop diuretics
    E. K$^+$ sparing diuretics
    F. Beta-blockers

    1. Blocks beta-receptors in the heart thus reducing heart rate and improving myocardial perfusion
    2. Causes negative inotropic effects which can be dangerous in some cases of heart failure
    3. Is a cause of delayed action potentials and may trigger ectopic beats
    4. Inhibits conversion of angiotensin I to angiotensin II, which is a vasoconstrictor, and through aldosterone promotes fluid reabsorption by the kidney
    5. Reduces fluid accumulation by increasing salt and water excretion
    6. Promotes fluid excretion and does not cause hypokalaemia
    7. Causes a dry cough or renal dysfunction
    8. Inhibits Na$^+$ pump in cardiac muscle thus increasing intracellular Ca^{2+}
    9. Increases ejection fraction and may cause regression of hypertrophy
    10. Increases vagal tone and slows conduction through the atrioventricular node

41. What effects do diuretics have on quality of life?

---

*MI, myocardial infarction; ACE, angiotensin-converting enzyme; AngII, angiotensin II

EXPLANATION: HEART FAILURE – TREATMENT OPTIONS

Treatment of HF is first to determine and treat the cause. If HF is due to chronic hypertension that should be managed initially (see appendix). If the problem is traced to a faulty valve (aortic stenosis or mitral regurgitation) then valve replacement should be considered. Ischaemia of the myocardium may also cause heart failure, which may benefit from Coronary Artery Bypass Graft (CABG) or balloon angioplasty.

The aims of drug treatment are to improve quality of life (increase exercise tolerance, decrease oedema), improve myocardial function and slow progression of failure.

1. **ACE inhibitors** (e.g. captopril, enalapril) block AngII formation and thus reduce vasoconstriction and increase water and salt excretion. This reduces preload, afterload, oedema and slows progression of disease. If dry cough develops due to breakdown of bradykinin, losartan (AngII inhibitor) can be given.
2. **Beta-blockers** (e.g. propanolol, metorolol) block beta-receptors in the heart, slowing HR and thus increasing myocardial perfusion. They are also shown to be very effective in slowing progression of myocyte dysfunction.
3. **Diuretics** (e.g. loop diuretics (frusemide), thiazide diuretics (bendrofluazide) or K^+ sparing (amiloride)) all work by increasing water and salt excretion and thus reducing oedema. They work in a variety of ways.
4. **Cardiac glycosides** (e.g. digoxin) inhibit Na^+ pump, which increases intracellular Ca^{2+} by reducing the effectiveness of Ca^{2+} transport out of cell at the end of depolarization. They increase contractility and improve function and may be used to treat arrhythmias. They are only used acutely as they increase myocardial work.

ACE inhibitors ⟶ increase salt + water excretion

reduces preload

dry cough (bradykinin)

Ang II inhibitor instead

Answers

40. 1 – F, 2 – F, 3 – C, 4 – A, 5 – D, 6 – E, 7 – A, 8 – F, 9 – F, 10 – C
41. They decrease shortness of breath, chest pain and prolong life, but increase frequency of micturation.

42. Case study

A 79-year-old man comes to see his GP and has the good fortune to meet you. He complains of chest discomfort on exertion and breathlessness. He has also had dizzy spells and felt as though he might faint a couple of times in the past week. On examination his blood pressure is 110/80 mmHg and his heart rate 82 bpm. His apex beat is displaced slightly and is thrusting. A soft ejection systolic murmur is appreciated radiating to the carotids. The second heart sound is softened. Carotid pulses are diminished.

    a. Explain the chest discomfort and dyspnoea upon exertion. Why does this man not suffer from orthopnoea or ankle swelling?

    b. Explain the episodes of dizziness

    c. Why is this man's jugular venous pressure not raised?

    d. Where is the murmur best heard?

    e. What is the likely diagnosis and what is the likely cause?

The patient was sent for an echocardiogram to assess the severity of the disease. It was decided that intervention was needed.

    f. Suggest a suitable treatment

43. Case study

A 63-year-old man suffered a myocardial infarction a few months ago. He now complains of dyspnoea, fatigue and has noticed palpitations. Upon careful history taking it becomes apparent that he also suffers from orthopnoea. On examination he has crackles bi-basally in his lungs and has a raised jugular venous pressure. His apex is displaced and is hyperdynamic. S1 is barely audible. A pansystolic murmur is appreciated, radiating to the apex.

    a. What is the valve most likely to be problematic?

    b. What is the likely mechanism behind the valvular problem, considering his recent myocardial infarction?

    c. Explain this man's symptoms.

    d. What is the next course of action?

    e. What intervention, if any, is required?

---

*LV, left ventricle; JVP, jugular venous pressure; BP, blood pressure; CO, cardiac output; MI, myocardial infarction

EXPLANATION: VALVE DISEASE

The most common cause of valve problems worldwide is rheumatic fever, causing both stenosis and regurgitation affecting any heart valves. Other causes include senile calcification (leading to stenosis), infective endocarditis (leading to regurgitation) and complications of MI and heart failure.

The most common cause of aortic valve disease is senile degeneration secondary to calcification causing stenosis. The murmur heard is best described diagrammatically.

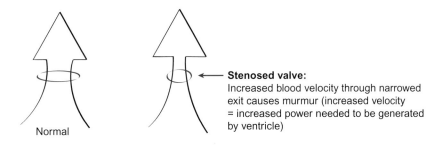

Normal

Stenosed valve:
Increased blood velocity through narrowed exit causes murmur (increased velocity = increased power needed to be generated by ventricle)

Think about the movement of blood. During systole the ventricles contract, increasing intraventricular pressure above that of the aorta and forcing the aortic valve to open. If this valve is 'stiff' it won't open so well and the heart has to pump harder to get the same volume of blood out. The murmur is heard due to the rush of blood through the narrowed valve, and is therefore best heard on the right sternal edge, 2nd intercostal space **(42d)** (see page 71).

As the man's heart hypertrophies in response to the increased effort at which it must now work, it gets larger and the **capillary density decreases** so angina is felt. Exertional dyspnoea and chest discomfort are an indication of LV failure, which may progress (see page 75). The right heart is not affected yet so JVP is not raised. Reduced carotid pulses, dizziness and low BP are a result of diminished CO (less blood can leave the heart through the narrowed valve).

Another common problem is **mitral regurgitation**. MI can involve and rupture the chordae tendinae or papillary muscles. This causes wild flailing of the valve leaflets. **Hypertrophy** can enlarge the atrioventricular passage and cause regurgitation, so even if the valve itself is intact it may not be large enough to fully close the passage. This causes **retrograde flow** through the atrioventricular passage as the ventricle contracts, heard as a pan (throughout) systolic murmur.

As blood is being pumped back into the atrium, pressure in the left atrium increases and is backed into the pulmonary system and then into the right heart. The increased work needed to pump against the increased pressure may cause heart failure (discussed on page 75).

An enlarged heart may be seen on chest X-ray. Echocardiography is the investigation of choice. Valve replacement surgery may be the only option (balloon valvuloplasty may help aortic stenosis).

Answers

42. See explanation
43. See explanation

44. Case study

A 2-year-old child is brought into the Emergency Department. He is small for his age and undernourished. He has a bluish tinge to his lips and is having trouble breathing. On examination the heart is enlarged and there is a harsh pansystolic murmur audible at the left sternal edge.

    a. Why is the infant struggling for breath? Comment on the significance of the blue tinge

    b. What are the possible causes of the murmur? Justify your answer

    c. Explain the mechanism of the infant's problem

45. Fallot's tetralogy is a congenital heart condition that consists of four separate defects. Which of the following statements are correct? Fallot's tetralogy consists of

    a. Ventricular and atrial septal defects, transposition of the great arteries and right ventricular hypertrophy

    b. Ventricular septal defect, pulmonary stenosis, overriding aorta and right ventricular hypertrophy

    c. Atrial septal defect, overriding aorta, right ventricular hypertrophy and patent ductus arteriosus

    d. Ventricular septal defect, pulmonary stenosis, aortic stenosis and right ventricular hypertrophy

46. Answer true or false for each of the following:

    a. Congenital coarctation of the aorta causes left ventricular failure

    b. An example of a right to left shunt is an atrial septal defect

    c. Transposition of the great arteries occurs when the left ventricle empties into the pulmonary artery and the right ventricle empties into the aorta

    d. Atrial septal defects are usually picked up during infancy

    e. Pulmonary vascular remodelling occurs when there is a long standing left to right shunt

*LV, left ventricle; RV, right ventricle; VSD, ventricular septal defect; ASD, atrial septal defect

EXPLANATION: CONGENITAL HEART ABNORMALITIES

To finish off this chapter here is a quick reminder about congenital heart abnormalities. The fetal circulation (dealt with on page 47) involves two right to left shunts bypassing the lungs and going straight into the systemic circulation. These should close at birth. After birth the systemic circulation is kept at a higher pressure than the pulmonary circulation, thus patent bypasses will become left to right shunts (i.e. the LV overpowers the RV). The same thing occurs with a VSD.

Long standing left to right shunts are a problem due to vascular remodelling. Shunting blood from the LV to RV causes LV and RV hypertrophy (as in heart failure due to mitral regurgitation) and causes pulmonary hypertension. Persistent pulmonary hypertension causes permanent changes (vascular remodelling). If it becomes so severe that pulmonary pressure exceeds systemic pressure the shunt will reverse, becoming a right to left shunt. This is where the cyanosis develops.

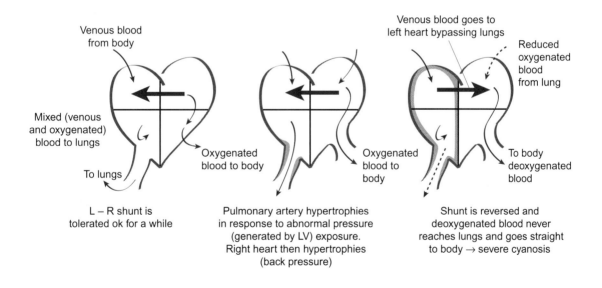

Venous blood from body

Mixed (venous and oxygenated) blood to lungs

To lungs

Oxygenated blood to body

L – R shunt is tolerated ok for a while

Pulmonary artery hypertrophies in response to abnormal pressure (generated by LV) exposure. Right heart then hypertrophies (back pressure)

Oxygenated blood to body

Venous blood goes to left heart bypassing lungs

Reduced oxygenated blood from lung

To body deoxygenated blood

Shunt is reversed and deoxygenated blood never reaches lungs and goes straight to body → severe cyanosis

Other problems include transposition of the great arteries in which the aorta and pulmonary artery are transposed, leading to severe central cyanosis causing death at two weeks, Fallot's tetralogy (which is a combination of RV hypertrophy leading to pulmonary stenosis, a VSD and an overriding aorta) and ASDs, not usually picked up until adulthood.

Answers
44. See explanation
45. b
46. T F T F T

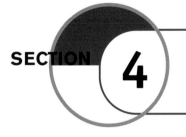

SECTION 4

THE PHYSIOLOGY OF CONDUCTION

THE PHYSIOLOGY OF CONDUCTION

1. Consider the nerve supply to the heart and answer true or false

a. The vagus nerve descends through the neck posterolateral to the common carotid arteries

b. The right recurrent laryngeal nerve arises from the right vagus nerve at the inferior border of the arch of the aorta

c. The right vagus nerve meets the left vagus nerve in the pulmonary and oesophageal plexuses

d. The vagus contributes sympathetic nerves to the cardiac plexus

e. Bronchial carcinoma may involve the left recurrent laryngeal nerve and consequently may affect the voice

2. Regarding the nerve supply to the heart

a. The cardiac plexus lies anterior to the bifurcation of the trachea and posterior to the arch of the aorta

b. The sympathetic supply comes from cervical and superior thoracic parts of the sympathetic trunks

c. The vagus supplies parasympathetic innervation responsible for an increase in heart rate

d. The cardiac plexus is responsible for control of heart rate, force of contraction and coronary artery dilation

e. The post-ganglionic nerve fibres from the cardiac plexus innervate the sinoatrial node and atrioventricular node

3. The SA node

a. Is a small collection of specialized myocytes responsible for initiating and regulating heart rate

b. Is located in the postero-inferior region of the interatrial septum, near the coronary sinus

c. Produces an impulse which spreads throughout the atrial myocardium

d. Produces an impulse that is conducted into the ventricles by the atrioventricular septum

e. Depolarizes over 100 times per minute

---

*SA node, sinoatrial node; AV node, atrioventricular node; HR, heart rate; SVC, superior vena cava

EXPLANATION: THE NERVOUS SUPPLY TO THE HEART

The cardiac plexus is responsible for higher input to the SA node and AV node. Parasympathetic nerves from the vagus (cranial nerve X) join sympathetic nerves from the cervical and upper thoracic sympathetic chain to form the cardiac plexus, which is sandwiched between the bifurcation of the trachea and the arch of the aorta. Nerves from this network innervate the SA node, AV node and coronary arteries.

Post-ganglionic sympathetic nerves cause an increase in the rate of depolarization of the SA node (and therefore HR), increase myocardial contractility and cause dilatation of the coronary arteries, i.e. everything needed for the heart to beat faster and harder.

Post-ganglionic parasympathetic (vagus) nerves have the opposite effect to the sympathetic system, but have no afferents to the myocardium so do not affect contractility.

Autonomic innervation of the heart is shown below:

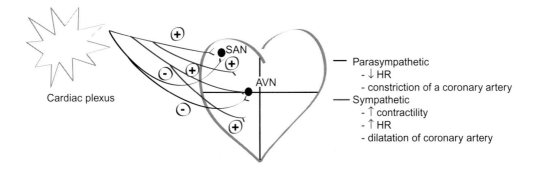

The SA node, located anterolaterally at the junction of the SVC and right atrium, initiates the impulse (about 70 per minute). The atrial impulse ends when it hits the atrioventricular septum which is non-conductive fibrous tissue (annulus fibrosus). The impulse is picked up by the AV node located in the interatrial septum.

Answers

1. T F F F T
2. T T F T T
3. T F T F F

4. Consider the AV node. Are the following statements true or false?

a. The atrioventricular node is smaller anatomically than the sinoatrial node
b. It produces a functionally significant delay of 1 s between contraction of the atria and ventricles
c. This functional delay corresponds to the PR interval on the electrocardiogram
d. Sympathetic stimulation decreases conduction velocity through the atrioventricular node and therefore increases the PR interval
e. The atrioventricular node is not capable of initiating ventricular beats by itself

5. Consider the bundle of His

a. It transfers impulses from the atrioventricular node through the annulus fibrosus
b. It splits into left and right bundle branches
c. The impulse jumps from the right to the left bundle branch
d. The left branch further divides into posterior and anterior fascicles
e. The bundle of His transmits the impulse to the Purkinje system which transmits the impulse to the rest of the myocardium

6. Choose from the following options to fill in the missing gaps in the paragraph below

Options

A. Ventricular myocardium
C. Sympathetic
E. Right
G. Sinoatrial node
I. Parasympathetic

B. Non-conducting
D. Cardiac plexus
F. Purkinje system
H. Left

Sympathetic and parasympathetic nerves form the **1** which innervates the **2** which is located anterolaterally at the junction of the SVC and right atrium. The impulse spreads across both atria until it reaches the annulus fibrosus which is located at the atrioventricular septum and is **3**. Here the AV node, located in the postero-inferior region of the interatrial septum, picks up the impulse. Ventricular rate can be increased by activation of **4** nerve fibres from the cardiac plexus. The impulse travels down the bundle of His and jumps from the **5** branch to the **6** branch. The left branch divides further into posterior and anterior fascicles. Depolarization of the septum occurs and the impulse is transmitted to the **7** which distributes the impulse and causes contraction of the **8**.

*SA node, sinoatrial node; AV node, atrioventricular node

EXPLANATION: SA AND AV NODES

Once the impulse from the SA node has been picked up by the AV node, a gap is needed (**~0.1 s**). Think about what is happening: the atria have just contracted, and therefore blood is moving from the atria to the respective ventricles. If the ventricles were to contract immediately then there would be no filling time and therefore no blood in the ventricles for the ventricles to pump out of the heart. The AV node has a very slow conduction time (0.05 m/s). Sympathetic stimulation from the cardiac plexus increases this conduction speed (therefore reducing conduction **time**) so the impulse is transmitted to the ventricles more quickly, facilitating a faster heart rate (by shortening of the PR interval). Parasympathetic stimulus has the opposite effect.

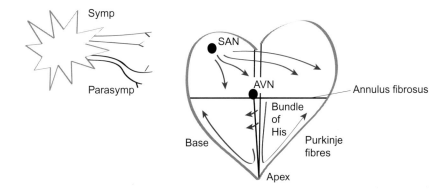

The impulse then leaves the AV node and travels down the interventricular septum, jumping from left to right bundle branches. Once the apex is reached, the Purkinje fibres distribute the impulse throughout the ventricular myocardium, causing the apex to contract first then the base (efficient pumping to get blood out).

Answers
4. T F T F F
5. T T F T T
6. 1 – D, 2 – G, 3 – B, 4 – C, 5 – H, 6 – E, 7 – F, 8 – A

7. **Consider action potentials in cardiac myocytes. Put these statements in the correct chronological order**

   A. An action potential is initiated and causes depolarization of myocytes (threshold value ~65 mV)
   B. When membrane potential falls to about −20 mV K$^+$ outward current becomes dominant, and rapid repolarization occurs
   C. The upstroke of the action potential reaches a positive value, limited by the existing outward K$^+$ current and inactivation of Na$^+$ channels
   D. At rest the membrane is most permeable to K$^+$ ions and the resting potential is dependent on the K$^+$ concentration gradient
   E. Membrane potential decays slowly over 250 ms due to Ca^{2+} channel activation resulting in an inward current
   F. Voltage-gated Na$^+$ channels are activated and the inward current caused overwhelms the existing outward K$^+$ current, and further depolarization occurs

8. **Examine the action potentials shown below (1–4). Match each one to the components of the conducting system of the heart below**

Options

A. Sinoatrial node
B. Atria
C. Atrioventricular node
D. Ventricles
E. Purkinje fibres

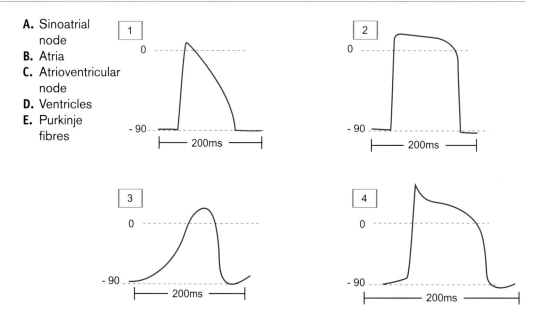

*AV node, atrioventricular node

EXPLANATION: CHANNELS AND DEPOLARIZATIONS

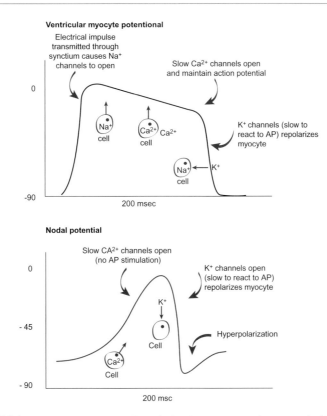

The above are helpful diagrams to memorize. Depolarization occurs, as in any excitable cell, by transmission of an electrical impulse. Myocytes form a syncytium through intercalated discs (see page 59). The action potential causes opening of Na^+ channels which causes depolarization of the membrane. In addition, this action potential also activates **voltage-sensitive L-type Ca^{2+} channels**, and these are slow to react. Therefore once the Na^+ permeability has returned to normal (and rapid repolarization would rapidly follow in skeletal muscle which is without type 2 Ca^{2+} channels), the slow vchannels open, and this produces another inward current to maintain the positive potential. K^+ channels are the slowest to react. Once the K^+ current becomes dominant as the Ca^{2+} current starts to decrease, rapid repolarization then occurs. Na^+ channels cannot be reactivated until their membrane potential becomes more negative than ~**65 mV**, thus giving rise to an absolute refractory period.

The action potential of a nodal cell is also shown here. There is no initiating electrical impulse and therefore no inward Na^+ current, so upstroke is due to slow Ca^{2+} current alone. This slower conduction is useful in the AV node (see page 87).

Answers

7. 1 – D, 2 – A, 3 – F, 4 – C, 5 – E, 6 – B
8. 1 – B, 2 – D, 3 – A or C, 4 – E

9. Consider the myocardium

a. Myocytes are connected via intercalated discs
b. The gap junctions in the region of an intercalated disc consist of proteins called connexons
c. The larger the gap junctions between cells, the faster the action potential spreads through the myocardium
d. Ischaemia of the myocardium may increase the resistance of gap junctions
e. The larger the size of the action potential, the slower the rate of conduction

10. With regard to electrical conduction through the heart

a. The P-wave recorded on an electrocardiogram represents depolarization of the left atrium only
b. The QRS complex, which represents ventricular depolarization, lasts 0.08 s
c. The S deflection represents atrial repolarization
d. The T-wave and the R-wave are both positive deflections because the wave of repolarization is in the same direction as the wave of depolarization
e. The ST segment represents isoelectric conditions in the myocardium, and means the ventricular mass is all depolarized

11. Consider the ECG

a. Tachycardia means a fast heart rate, and the QRS complex is shortened as a result
b. The PR interval is the time the action potential is held up in the atrioventricular node
c. The PR interval varies between 0.12 and 0.2 s
d. A QRS complex of greater duration than 0.08 s may be pathological
e. In health, a QRS complex is always preceded by a P-wave

*ECG, electrocardiogram; AV node; atrioventricular node

EXPLANATION: ELECTRICAL CONDUCTION IN THE HEART

The ECG measures the wave of **electrical conduction** through the myocardium in a particular direction (see page 93). The key to understanding ECGs is to know which way the wave of depolarization spreads through the myocardium. The example below is lead II, which looks straight through the middle of the heart.

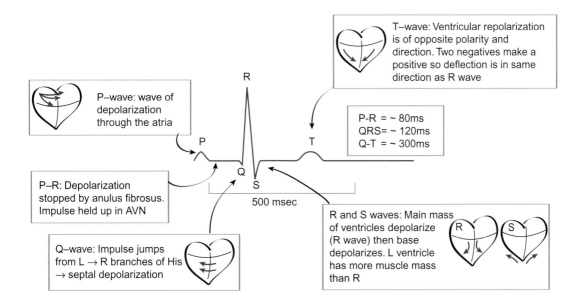

Remember that the repolarization of both atria occurs during ventricular depolarization so is masked by the larger wave. Repolarization waves are of **opposite polarity** and **direction** and so the deflection appears in the same direction as the depolarization (i.e. two negatives make a positive).

The QRS complex (systole) is fixed and does not change in duration. However as heart rate increases, sympathetic stimulation of the AV node causes a decrease in conduction time so the PR interval shortens. This allows more complete cycles in a given time period (an increase in heart rate).

Answers
9. T T F T F (see page 59)
10. F T F F T
11. F T T T T

12. **Choose leads from the list of options below and put in the correct position according to which direction is measured through the heart**

Options

A. aVF   **B.** aVR

C. aVL   **D.** Lead I

E. Lead II   **F.** Lead III

13. **Answer true or false for each of the following about ECGs**

   a. The electrocardiogram is based around Einthoven's triangle, the points of which are approximated by the limb leads

   b. The bipolar leads measure the potential difference between two limb leads

   c. There are eight chest leads used in common clinical practice

   d. Ischaemia of the myocardium cannot be detected on a standard electrocardiogram

   e. Acute changes during a myocardial infarction are sometimes seen as an ST segment elevation

*ECG, electrocardiogram

EXPLANATION: ECG LEADS

Now that you know the path that the conduction wave takes through the myocardium, you are able to draw any ECG trace given the direction that the lead is looking at. Consider the spread of depolarization through the myocardium. The ECG measures the resultant vector from the addition of all imagined vectors representing the spread of depolarization.

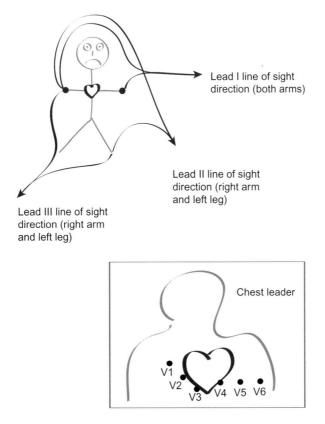

The classic bipolar leads are obtained by measuring the potential difference between two limbs. For example, lead II measures the voltage between the right arm and left leg (i.e. straight through the centre of the heart). Unipolar leads are obtained by using one limb electrode and measuring the voltage against an estimation of zero, obtained by connecting the remaining limb leads together by a resistor. These leads measure between one point of Einthoven's triangle and the centre, as shown below. In addition there are six chest (unipolar) leads that provide anterior views of the heart.

Answers

12. 1 – C, 2 – D, 3 – E, 4 – A, 5 – F, 6 – B
13. T T F F T

14. Examine the ECGs below and match with the most appropriate description from the following list

Options

A. Sinus tachycardia
B. Normal electrocardiogram
C. First degree heart block
D. Ischaemic heart disease
E. Myocardial infarction
F. Second degree heart block

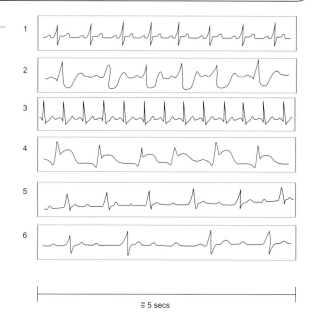

1

2

3

4

5

6

≅ 5 secs

15. Classify the arrhythmias listed below into one of the two following groups: (1) supraventricular arrhythmia or (2) ventricular arrhythmia

Options

A. Atrial fibrillation
B. Ventricular fibrillation
C. Ventricular tachycardia
D. Sinus tachycardia
E. Atrial flutter

16. For the arrhythmias listed in question 19, match the mechanism of arrhythmia with one of the specific arrhythmias listed below

1. Elevated sympathetic tone
2. Re-entry arrhythmia associated with MI and ischaemia
3. Dilated atrium causing multiple re-entry currents
4. Loss of cardiac output due to galloping ventricular rhythm

*ECG, electrocardiogram; HR, heart rate; MI, myocardial infarction; AV node, atrioventricular node

EXPLANATION: READING AN ECG

ECG reading is all about pattern recognition. Become familiar with the trends shown in question 15. An HR over 100 bpm is called a **tachycardia**. Sinus tachycardia means that every ventricular depolarization (QRS complex) is preceded by a P-wave (atrial depolarization) and thus the conduction pathway is working correctly, if a little on the fast side. In heart block (**bradycardia**), QRS complexes are sometimes missed, for example two P-waves per QRS complex may be seen, indicating a problem with the conduction pathway.

In ischaemic heart disease ST segment **depression** is classically seen. During an MI, ST segment **elevation** is sometimes seen, and inversion of the T-wave (demonstrating abnormal repolarization due to delayed conduction as a result of scar tissue) may be seen during the MI and post MI.

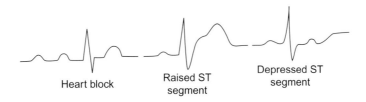

Heart block   Raised ST   Depressed ST
                    segment   segment

Arrhythmias may develop along any part of the conduction pathway. If they develop before the bundle of His they are called supraventricular arrhythmias/tachycardias. Arrhythmias below the bundle of His (i.e. originating in the ventricles) are called ventricular arrhythmias. **Ventricular arrhythmias** are far more dangerous as it is the ventricular rate and function that determines cardiac output. **Atrial fibrillation** is quite common in the elderly and well tolerated (but ventricular fibrillation is often fatal). This is because the AV node has the ability to 'filter out' atrial noise, and even to set its own rhythm so the ventricles beat at a reasonable pace.

Answers

14. 1 – B, 2 – D, 3 – A, 4 – E, 5 – C, 6 – F
15. Supraventricular – A, D, E; ventricular – B, C
16. 1 – D, 2 – C, 3 – A, 4 – B

17. With regard to the mechanism of arrhythmias which of the following statements are true?

    a. Early after depolarizations occur during the repolarization phases of the action potential
    b. Early after depolarizations are more common during tachycardia
    c. Blockade of K^+ current may cause early after depolarizations by increasing action potential duration
    d. Quinidine is a drug that suppresses the K^+ current
    e. Class IC and III drugs increase action potential duration and hence predispose to early after depolarizations

18. True or false? Concerning the mechanism of arrhythmia generation

    a. Delayed after depolarizations are caused by excessive Na^+ load in the myocyte
    b. Digitalis toxicity is a known inducer of delayed after depolarization arrhythmia
    c. Shorter action potentials predispose to delayed after depolarizations
    d. Enhancing the transient inward current caused by Na^+ increases the likelihood of developing a delayed after depolarization
    e. Delayed and early after depolarizations are examples of impulse generation abnormalities

19. With regard to the mechanism of arrhythmia generation

    a. Myocytes outside the conduction system normally spontaneously depolarize
    b. Ischaemia can increase the automaticity of myocytes by reducing membrane potential
    c. Hypokalaemia decreases the automaticity of myocytes
    d. Catecholamines have no effect on automaticity of myocytes
    e. An electrocardiogram demonstrates variations in the heart rate

20. With regard to the mechanism of arrhythmia formation

    a. Re-entry arrhythmias occur when an impulse is delayed in one area of the heart and then excites areas already excited by other, non-delayed impulses
    b. A unidirectional block is essential
    c. A central unexcitable region must be present, such as scar tissue
    d. Slowed conduction occurs as a result of elongated phase 2 (plateau) phase
    e. Re-entry arrhythmias are caused by class IC drugs

*EAD, early after depolarization; DAD, delayed after depolarization; SA node, sinoatrial node; AV node, atrioventricular node; MI, myocardial infarction

EXPLANATION: ARRHYTHMIAS

Re-entry arrhythmias are a defect in conduction whereas EADs and DADs are defects in initiation of impulse. Myocytes outside the SA node and AV node may start to spontaneously depolarize. The **automaticity** (= ability to spontaneously depolarize) of myocytes is increased by ischaemia, hypokalaemia, fibre stretch and catecholamines. In addition, oscillations in the membrane potential following depolarizations may occur. **EADs** occur during the terminal plateau or repolarization phase (page 89). These are likely to develop during episodes of hypokalaemia or bradycardia, and cause torsade de pointes arrhythmias. Agents that prolong the action potential or increase the inward current predispose to these types of arrhythmia. Similarly **DADs** are also caused by agents that prolong the action potential. However these are caused by excessive $[Ca^{2+}]$ in myocytes which cause a transient inward current (caused by Na^+ entry due to the $3Na^+ - Ca^{2+}$ exchanger) (page 61). Remember that ischaemia causes the gap junctions between myocytes to dissociate and causes prolonged conduction time, lengthening action potentials and predisposing to arrhythmia.

For re-entry arrhythmias to initiate, all of the following have to be present

- Central inexciatable region, e.g. scar tissue after MI
- Zone of slowed conduction
- Unidirectional block.

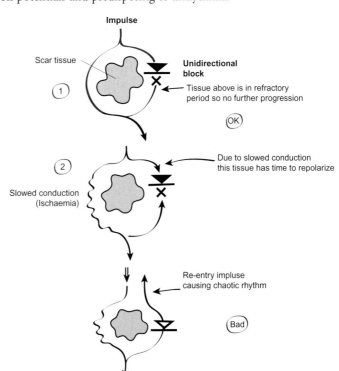

An impulse with reduced conduction speed, thus allowing the myocardium to recover from its refractive period, may recirculate around the scar tissue and through the unidirectional block in the wrong direction. Thus the impulse wave may circulate around the scar tissue, causing multiple action potentials.

Answers
17. T F T T T
18. F T F T T
19. F T F F T
20. T T T F T

21. Case study

A 70-year-old man with known hypertension and diabetes is brought into the Emergency Department complaining of shortness of breath made worse on lying down. He has no chest pain, but on examination his HR was found to be 150 and basal crackles were auscultated in both lungs. An ECG was ordered (shown below).

  a. Name two other standard tests that you would perform to help reach a diagnosis
  b. Describe the electrocardiogram appearance. Comment on rate, rhythm and any abnormalities that may be present

From Houghton, A., Gray, D., *Making Sense of the ECG*, 2nd edn, Arnold 2003.

  c. Name a possible diagnosis and justify your answer. What underlying pathology may have caused the abnormality?
  d. What is causing the man's shortness of breath?
  e. What is the main concern associated with this problem?
  f. What would be your choice of treatment?
  g. Name the four main classes of drugs and their mode of action. Give an example for each one

The man returns two years later. He presents with flaccid hemiplegia, and sensory loss on the same side.
  h. What is the likely diagnosis?
  i. What might have caused this?

*HR, heart rate; ECG, electrocardiogram; MI, myocardial infarction; AV node, atrioventricular node

EXPLANATION: ATRIAL FIBRILLATION CASE STUDY

This is a very common complaint clinically, so get used to it now. Taking a careful history helps. No chest pain suggests against an MI. The high HR and the bi-basal crackles suggestive of pulmonary oedema secondary to heart failure needs investigating. An ECG is done immediately as is a chest X-ray (to look for an enlarged heart) and blood tests (to look for cardiac enzymes and thyroid function). An echocardiogram may be organized later. The ECG opposite shows a rate of around 150, however it is **irregularly irregular**. There are no distinct P-waves. This is the typical appearance seen in **atrial fibrillation**.

Atrial rhythm can be 300–600 bpm but the AV node only responds intermittently, hence the irregular ventricular rate. Atrial fibrillation can be idiopathic or be caused by heart failure, hypertension, MI, mitral valve disease, etc. Shortness of breath is due to pulmonary congestion secondary to impaired ventricular function and back pressure into the pulmonary system (see page 75).

Atrial fibrillation is well tolerated but stasis of blood in the atria increases the risk of thrombus formation (as does smoking and diabetes mellitus), therefore the patient should be given **anticoagulants**, such as warfarin or aspirin.

Cardioversion is the treatment of choice, and this can be done medically (amiodarone) or by using DC cardioversion. Initial slowing of the ventricular rate (important as patients with compromised coronary flow may start to experience ischaemic pain due to reduced time for myocardial perfusion – remember phasic flow!) are beta-blockers, digoxin and Ca^{2+}-channel blockers, all of which slow AV node conduction (see page 101 and appendix).

Atrial fibrillation is often a chronic problem and cardioversion sometimes does not prevent a reccurrence. In this man's case atrial fibrillation reoccurred, and an embolus formed in the atria and ended up in the cerebral circulation, causing stroke.

Answers

21. See explanation

22. Answer true or false for each of the following

a. Supraventricular tachycardia originates above the atrioventricular node
b. Atrial fibrillation is caused by chaotic depolarizations of the sinoatrial node
c. Ventricular tachycardia and ventricular fibrillation are the same phenomenon
d. Ventricular fibrillation may cause death due to reduced cardiac output
e. Underlying heart disease is usually present to precipitate an arrhythmia

23. Answer the following with true or false

a. A broad QRS complex is seen in junctional tachycardia
b. A broad QRS complex is seen in atrial fibrillation
c. A broad QRS complex is seen in ventricular fibrillation
d. Broad complex tachycardias are life threatening
e. Treatment of choice is defibrillation

24. With regard to Wolff–Parkinson–White tachycardia, which of the following statements are true?

a. It is a congenital defect
b. There is an increased risk of tachyarrhythmia
c. The condition improves as the infant matures
d. Surgery is not an option
e. The ECG in a patient with WPW syndrome is completely normal

25. Answer true or false for each of the following

a. Bradycardia is defined as a heart rate of less than 60 bpm
b. Bradycardia is due to a failure of the atrioventricular node but the rest of the conduction pathway is normal
c. Bradycardia is never seen post myocardial infarction
d. Heart block can present with episodes of fainting or dizziness
e. Atropine is given to cure this condition

*WPW, Wolff–Parkinson–White; AV node, atrioventricular node; HR, heart rate; CO, cardiac output; MI, myocardial infarction; SA node, sinoatrial node

EXPLANATION: MORE ARRHYTHMIAS

Broad complex arrhythmias originate **below** the AV node (i.e. in the ventricles) and are life threatening. If an impulse arrives in the ventricles via the AV node the QRS complex will be narrow (therefore all other tach-yarrhythmias are narrow complex arrhythmias). The exception is Wolff–Parkinson–White syndrome, which is a junctional tachcardia and has a broad QRS of specific appearance (see below).

Opposite is a diagram representing the three most common types of **junctional** tachycardia. Page 103 discusses other causes of tachycardia such as atrial fibrillation and re-entry arrhythmia (see also page 99).

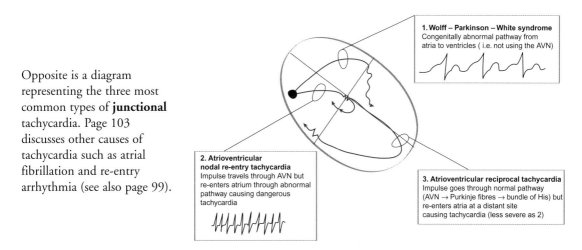

1. Wolff – Parkinson – White syndrome
Congenitally abnormal pathway from atria to ventricles (i.e. not using the AVN)

2. Atrioventricular nodal re-entry tachycardia
Impulse travels through AVN but re-enters atrium through abnormal pathway causing dangerous tachycardia

3. Atrioventricular reciprocal tachycardia
Impulse goes through normal pathway (AVN → Purkinje fibres → bundle of His) but re-enters atria at a distant site causing tachycardia (less severe as 2)

Bradycardia is the slowing of the HR below 60 bpm. The worry is that if this is maintained the body does not receive adequate CO and cardiac failure (and multi-organ failure) will follow. The problem can be in any part of the conduction system:

- **SA node** (e.g. sick sinus syndrome in which the SA node is involved during an MI and fails to depolarize properly leading to a drastic fall in HR)
- **AV node** (AV heart block in which slowing of the conduction impulse that normally occurs in the AV node is excessive and impulses travelling through the AV node may be lost and never transmitted to the ventricles)
- **Bundle of His** (bundle branch block, which causes delayed contraction of either the right or the left ventricle)
- **Others** (such as hypothermia, hypothyroidism, drugs or acute ischaemia of the myocardium)

The management is to treat the underlying cause. Atropine can temporarily increase HR, but external pacing may be needed.

Answers
22. T F F T T
23. F F T T T
24. T T F F F
25. T F F T F

26. Match the class of drug with its principal mechanism of action labelled 1–5. You may use an answer more than once or not at all

Options:

A. Class IA   B. Class IB
C. Class IC   D. Class II
E. Class IV   F. Class III

1. Blocks beta-receptors   2. Blocks Ca^{2+} channels
2. Blocks Na^+ channels   4. Acts on nodal tissue
5. Acts on the myocardium   6. Blocks K^+ channels

27. Case study

An elderly man is brought into the Emergency Department unconscious. An ECG is performed. It is shown below (1)

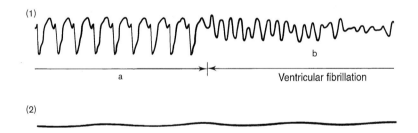

From Houghton, A., Gray, D., *Making Sense of the ECG*, 2nd edn, Arnold 2003.

a. Is this typical of a supraventricular tachycardia? Explain your answer
b. Would you expect a cardiac output from this patient (i.e. any carotid pulses)? Explain your answer
c. What would be your first choice of treatment? If unsuccessful what would you resort to?
d. After treatment the patient's ECG looks like (2). Would you continue treatment? Explain your answer

*ECG, electrocardiogram; SVT, supraventricular tachycardia

EXPLANATION: MANAGEMENT OF ARRHYTHMIAS

The diagram below shows the origin of some common arrhythmias.

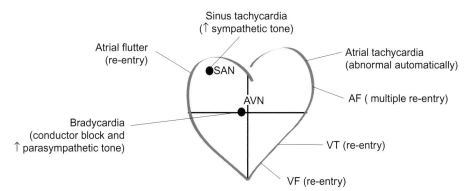

Treatment is decided based on the underlying reason for the arrhythmia. A brief guide is shown below.

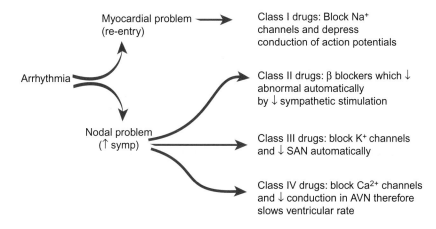

The man in the case study is in ventricular tachycardia (a) (which appears as a broad QRS complex on the ECG, compared with a narrow complex associated with SVTs). The ventricular rate is ~300 bpm and so the diastolic time is not long enough to allow filling of the ventricles and there is reduced or no output (no pulses). This pattern can easily progress to **ventricular fibrillation** (b) (ventricular contraction is disorganized and there is no output). First, you would try pharmacological cardioversion (amiodarone, digoxin) and if that does not work, defibrillation to restart the heart in sinus rhythm. If the patient reaches **asystole** (c) ('no contraction phase') (ECG 2) there is no electrical activity present and therefore there is no point continuing with defibrillation. Atropine may help if P-waves are still present.

Answers
26. 1 – D, 2 – E, 3 – A, B, C, 4 – D, E, F, 5 – A, B, C, 6 – F
27. See explanation

OVERVIEW OF THE CARDIOVASCULAR DRUGS

PHARMACOLOGY OF HYPERTENSION (PAGES 9 AND 21)

Hypertension causes heart failure, coronary artery disease, stroke and renal failure, therefore it is important to control it!

Diuretics

- **Loop diuretics (frusemide)** Increases Na^+ and water excretion from ascending loop of Henle by blocking the $Na^+/K^+/2Cl^-$ co-transporter. Used for mild heart failure and blood pressure control. Causes hypokalaemia and arrythmias
- **Thiazide diuretic (bendrofluazide)** Blocks the Na^+/Cl^- co-transporter in the distal convoluted tubule and collecting duct of kidney, therefore reducing reabsorption of water. Used to treat hypertension and mild heart failure. Causes hypokalaemia and arrhythmias
- **K+ sparing (spirolactone)** Blocks aldosterone from binding to receptor therefore reducing Na reabsorption and causing water, Na^+ and Cl^- excretion. Weak, as only 2 per cent of Na^+ reabsorption is under aldosterone control. Can cause hyperkalaemia. Often used in combination with others

Beta–blockers

- **Beta 1/beta 2 (propanolol)** Antagonize beta-receptors non-selectively, causing decrease in cardiac output and blood pressure (cardiac output subsequently returns to normal, leaving blood pressure lowered). Also used to treat arrhythmia, myocardial infarction and angina. Causes peripheral problems by acting on beta 2-receptors (cold hands, muscle aches). **Never give to asthmatics!**
- **Beta 1-selective (atenolol/metoprolol)** Selective beta 1 receptor blockade has less peripheral side effects but **never give to asthmatics!**

Calcium channel blockers

- **Nifedipine/amlodipine** Inhibits L-type Ca^{2+} channels in smooth and cardiac muscle. Reduced calcium means reduced contraction, therefore peripheral resistance decreased

ACE inhibitors

- **Captopril/enalapril** Vasodilation by inhibiting formation of angiotensin II (vasoconstrictor). Angiotensin II also activates aldosterone (responsible for Na^+ and water reabsorption) so therefore increased excretion leading to decreased PR. Also decreased left ventricular remodelling in left ventricular fibrillation

Angiotensin II receptor antagonists

- **Losartan** Those who have a dry cough with ACE inhibitors (due to reduced bradykinin breakdown) can have AII receptor antagonists

PHARMACOLOGY OF THROMBOSIS (PAGES 25, 27 AND 43)

Anticoagulants

- **Heparin** Activates antithrombin III and inhibits clotting factors IIa, IXa–XIVa, and thus stops the formation of fibrin which stops clot formation. Used for acute arterial and venous thrombosis. Works in minutes. Protamine sulphate counteracts effects
- **Warfarin** Vitamin K antagonist forming ineffective clotting factors VII, IX, X and prothrombin. Takes days to work. If bleeding occurs (warfarin poisoning) then give vitamin K or clotting factors

Fibrolytic drugs

- **Streptokinase** Activates plasminogen and increases plasmin formation which breaks down fibrin, breaking down the clot. May cause bleeding (e.g. stroke). Can only be used once in a lifetime due to allergic sensitization
- **Tissue plasminogen activators** (**alteplase**) Clot-sensitive proteases that specifically activate plasminogen bound to fibrin. More expensive so used less frequently. May cause bleeding

Antiplatelet drugs

- **Aspirin** Prophylaxis against clot formation. Inhibits cyclo-oxygenase (COX) and therefore reduced synthesis of thromboxane A_2, so reducing platelet activation, adhesion and aggregation

PHARMACOLOGY OF ANGINA (PAGE 39)

Nitrates

- **Glyceryl trinitrate (GTN)** $R\text{-}O\text{-}NO_2$ structure works by causing nitric oxide to be released, which increases cyclic guanosine monophosphate (cGMP), decreases Ca^{2+} and causes smooth muscle relaxation in coronary arteries (and peripheral arteries) causing increased blood flow to the myocardium and decreased central venous pressure, leading to decreased oxygen demand on the heart

Ca^{2+} channel blockers

- **Nifedipine/verapamil** Block Ca^{2+} entry into cells, therefore reduced force production and reduced oxygen demand. Verapamil works principally on the heart and nifedipine works mainly on smooth muscle in the periphery and coronary arteries (vasodilatation)

K^+-ATP channel activators

- **Nicorandil** Opens ATP-sensitive ion channels in vasculature and cardiac muscle cells causing hyperpolarization thus vasodilatation and decreased total peripheral resistance

Beta-blockers

- **Atenolol** See above. Decreases force of contraction (therefore decreased O_2 demand) and decreases heart rate (decreased O_2 demand and increased O_2 supply from coronary (phasic) flow)

PHARMACOLOGY OF HEART FAILURE (PAGE 77)

ACE inhibitors

- **Captopril/enalapril** Blocks formation of angiotensin II, thus decreasing total peripheral resistance and reducing water volume (reducing amount of aldosterone present) and reducing oedema. Improves exercise tolerance and slows progression of heart failure

Diuretics

- **Frusemide/bendrofluazide/spirolactone** See above. Used to treat patients with fluid retention (oedema) and improve symptoms of shortness of breath and ankle swelling associated with heart failure

Beta-blockers

- **Propanolol/atenolol** See above. Decrease symptoms of heart failure and reduce cardiac remodelling. Reduce mortality. Decrease sympathetic stimulus to remodelling

Inotropic drugs

- **Cardiac glycosides** (digoxin) Cause a reduction in calcium passage out of the myocyte after contraction has occurred by inhibiting Na^+/K^+ exchanger. More Ca^{2+} in the cell causes a greater force to be produced by the myocyte. May cause delayed action depolarization. Also decrease atrioventricular node conduction by increasing vagal stimulation. Increase mortality if used long term due to toxicity
- **Beta 1 adrenoreceptor agonists** (dobutamine) Increase adenylate cyclase activity which increases cAMP and causes an increase in heart rate and force to improve cardiac output. May increase mortality if used long term

PHARMACOLOGY OF ARRHYTHMIA (PAGES 99 AND 101)

Antiarrhythmics

- **Class IA drugs** (quinidone) All class I drugs act by blocking Na^+ channels and slowing down conduction in the myocardium. They also interrupt re-entry pathways by converting a unidirectional block into a bi-directional block. IA drugs increase refractory period. May cause nausea and vomiting
- **Class IB drugs** (lidocaine) Specifically block Na^+ channels in abnormal myocardium which is depolarized/high frequency depolarizing tissue. Used for treating ventricular fibrillation and ventricular tachycardia

- **Class IC drugs** (flecainide) Depress conduction in normal and depolarized myocardium. Useful for blocking re-entry pathways
- **Class II drugs** (propanolol) Beta-blockers. Decrease beta-adrenoreceptor-mediated Ca^{2+} conductance and tachycardia. Used for blockade in nodal tissue thus used to treat supraventricular tachycardia/ventricular tachycardia post myocardial infarction
- **Class III drugs** (amiodarone) Block K^+ channels and increase both action potential duration and refractory time, leading to a decrease in heart rate. Also inhibit sinoatrial node automaticity. Excellent cardioverters. Used for treating all arrhythmias, but sometimes use is contraindicated
- **Class IV drugs** (verapamil) Block Ca^{2+} channels and therefore decrease conduction velocity and increase refractory period in the atrioventricular node. Slower conduction in atrioventricular node leads to decreased ventricular rate. Good for supraventricular tachycardia

GLOSSARY

Acetylcholine (ACh)	Neurotransmitter released at parasympathetic nerve endings
Adenosine triphosphate (ATP)	The battery of the cell. When ATP is split into ADP + P_i, energy is released and used by the cell. Adenosine diphosphate (ADP) is reattached to P_i in mitochondria (recharging)
Adrenaline	Neurotransmitter released by sympathetic nerve endings
Antidiuretic peptide (antidiuretic hormone (ADH) or vasopressin)	Peptide released by the posterior pituitary which acts on the collecting ducts of the kidney and results in an increase in water reabsorption
Aortic valve (AV)	Valve found in the left side of the heart at the root of the aorta. It guards the outflow of the left ventricle
Atrial fibrillation	Irregularly irregular heart rhythm caused by disrupted atrial myocardium
Atrial naturetic peptide (ANP)	Released from atrial myocytes when they are stretched due to increased blood volume. Causes raised glomerular filtration rate by kidneys and decreased renin (thus less Na^+ and water retention)
Atrioventricular node (AV node)	Specialized cardiac tissue which transmits and modifies the electrical impulse of the heart from the atria to the ventricles
Blood pressure (BP)	Measured as systolic pressure/diastolic pressure
Cardiac output (CO)	The stroke volume multiplied by the heart rate. Measured in mL/min
Central venous pressure (CVP)	Measure of how well the heart is coping. A high CVP indicates the heart is struggling to move blood on to the arterial system, hence more blood is left in the venous system
Chronic obstructive pulmonary disease (COPD)	Chronic lung condition which shows an irreversible obstructive picture, and may lead to pulmonary hypertension and right heart failure (cor pulmonale). Largely caused by smoking
Computer tomography (CT) scan	A scanning technique able to reconstruct multiple X-ray images into three-dimensional cross-section or sagittal views of the body
Contractility	Ability of cardiac muscle to produce force, independently of any change in fibre length. Related to intracellular Ca^{2+}. Inotropic agents such as noradrenaline and digoxin, or an increase in heart rate, all increase intracellular Ca^{2+} and therefore increase contractility.
Deep vein thrombosis (DVT)	Clot of blood stuck in the deep vein system of a leg, causing unilateral leg swelling
Electrocardiogram (ECG)	Measures electrical activity in the heart at various views. It is altered when conduction through the heart is pathological
End diastolic pressure (EDP)	Pressure in a chamber of the heart at the end of the diastolic phase (relaxation)
End diastolic volume (EDV)	Volume of blood in a chamber of the heart at the end of the diastolic phase (relaxation)
End systolic volume (ESV)	Volume of blood left in a chamber of the heart at the end of the systolic phase (contraction)
Haemoglobin (Hb)	Protein found in red blood cells that binds oxygen at the lungs and releases it at the tissues

Heart failure	Can be right sided (RHF), left sided (LHF) or congestive (CHF). The heart is unable to produce an adequate cardiac output to perfuse the tissues, or can do so only with an elevated EDP
Heart rate (HR)	Measured in beats per minute (bpm)
High density lipoprotein (HDL)	Fat found in the diet and produced by liver. 'Good fat'
Jugular venous pressure (JVP)	Pulsation in the neck seen when the right side of the heart is under strain or there is pulmonary hypertension
Low density lipoprotein (LDL)	Fat found in the diet, and produced by the liver. Responsible for the formation of atheromatous plaques
Mitral valve (MV)	Valve found in the left side of the heart between the atrium and the ventricle
Myocardial infarction (MI)	Part of the myocardium becomes necrotic and dies following a failure of the coronary circulation to supply the muscle with oxygen
Nitric oxide (NO)	Formerly known as endothelium-derived relaxing factor, it is released by the endothelium and causes smooth muscle relaxation. It is also used in the treatment of angina
Noradrenaline	Neurotransmitter released by sympathetic nerve endings
Prostacyclin (PGI$_2$)	Released by the endothelium, it causes smooth muscle relaxation
Prostaglandin H$_2$ (PGH$_2$)	Released by the endothelium, it causes vasoconstriction in times of injury to minimise blood loss
Pulmonary embolism (PE)	Blood clot stuck in the pulmonary system causing V/Q mismatching. Life threatening
Red blood cells (RBCs)	Haemoglobin-containing cells with no nucleus specifically designed to carry oxygen from the lungs to the peripheral tissues
Sarcoplasmic reticulum (SR)	Vesicles or tubules found in striated muscle. Responsible for the transmission of electrical impulses and storage (and release) of calcium
Sinoatrial node (SA node)	The initiator of the electrical impulse that causes myocardial contraction
Starling's Law	Change in force generation due to a change in initial fibre length in the myocyte. The more pressure the myocyte is under (due to more blood in the compartment), the greater the fibre stretch and the greater the force generated
Superior vena cava (SVC)	The large vein draining blood from the head, neck and arms into the right side of the heart (right atrium)
Supraventricular tachycardia (SVT)	Tachycardia that originates from the AV node, the atria or the SA node
Thromboxane A$_2$ (TXA$_2$)	Released by the endothelium, it causes vasoconstriction
Ventricular fibrillation	Irregular, wide complex ventricular rhythm caused by serious disease of the ventricular myocardium. Life threatening
Voltage-operated calcium channels (VOCC)	Found in membranes of muscle cells, they are opened by an electrical impulse, allowing calcium into the cell, which is needed for the contraction process

INDEX